"*The Science of Sitting* is clear and concise enough to read in one sitting and comprehensive enough to inform you that you shouldn't. This is an excellent review of the postural contribution to the pathology that keeps most doctors in business."
Thomas A. McClure, M.D., Board-Certified Occupational Medicine Specialist, Medical Director CPMC Occupational Health Services

"This book contains good-to-know and in-depth information on ergonomics. It describes the workings of the human spine and shows how a proper posture can improve productivity and performance in any workplace. As an ergonomics specialist, I find this book to be very informative and written in a style that is easy to understand for everyone."
Joe Lezada, C.A.E., Ergonomics Specialist, Health Plan of San Mateo

"Dr. Carb uses common everyday language to explain the value of, and guidelines for, healthy sitting posture for application at work or home."
Sally A. Shute, M.A., C.I.E., C.E.E.S., Ergonomics Consultant, Bureau Veritas

No project w   : the friendly
cooperation   anks to the
above peer r   hinen, M.D.,
for their valu

Posture matters.

In this competitive world it helps to differentiate yourself and make a positive first impression when interviewing, making presentations, attending events, or even when finding a mate...

Body language speaks loudly.

Good posture says youth, health, attention, confidence, strength, and success. Bad posture says just the opposite.

Your posture becomes you.

A connection exists between your body's frame and your frame of mind. Your posture reflects not only the position you are most often in, but also how you see yourself—which is part of how other people see you.

The Science of Sitting

Made Simple

How to look and feel better with good posture in ten easy steps

The Science of Sitting

Made Simple

How to look and feel better with good posture in ten easy steps

Gregg J. Carb, D.C., C.A.E.

First Edition

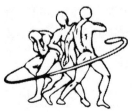

Posture Press - San Francisco, California
www.scienceofsitting.com

The Science of Sitting Made Simple
How to look and feel better with good posture in ten easy steps

Copyright © 2008 Gregg J. Carb

Author: Gregg J. Carb, D.C., C.A.E.
Editor: Elizabeth Bales-Stutes
Illustrators: Rich Sigberman
                     Yan Ling Li
Graphics/Layout: Shirley Situ, Imagink

Published by Posture Press – www.posturepress.com
220 Sansome St. #530
San Francisco, CA 94104 U.S.A.
First Edition
ISBN 978-0-9716020-5-2
Printed in the United States
Library of Congress Control Number 2008920176

Publisher's Cataloging-in-Publication Data

Carb, Gregg J.
       The science of sitting made simple : how to look and
   feel better with good posture in ten easy steps / Gregg
   J. Carb. -- 1st ed.
       p. cm.
       LCCN 2008920176
       ISBN-13: 978-0-9716020-5-2
       ISBN-10: 0-9716020-5-0

       1. Posture. 2. Sitting position. 3. Back--Care and
   hygiene.   I. Title.

   RA781.5.C37 2008   613.7'8
                          QBI08-600052

CONTENTS

List of Illustrations   x

Preface   xiii
The swan and the ducklings

Dear Reader   xv
Disclaimer and advice

Introduction   17
Why posture is important and what this book will
help you accomplish

STEP ONE   21
Understanding Your Spine's Normal Shape
Explains the normal shape of the spine, its purpose,
and its parts

STEP TWO   27
Keeping It Together
Covers the role soft tissues play in holding the spine
together

STEP THREE   31
Learning How You Get Bent out of Shape
Reviews the effect poor posture has on the shape
of the spine

STEP FOUR   35
Understanding How Degeneration Happens
Details the process of wear and tear in a spine that
is bent out of shape

STEP FIVE   39
Understanding Your Correct Posture
Demonstrates neutral posture and the natural
forward contour of the lower spine

STEP SIX   47
Sitting up When You Sit Down
Discusses the basics of sitting correctly

STEP SEVEN   59
Using Your Awareness to Stop Slumping
Clarifies the importance of increasing your posture
awareness to stop slumping

STEP EIGHT   67
Undoing Damage with Extension Stretching
Shows how to perform a stretch to help overcome
tight muscles and to reverse slumping

STEP NINE   73
Moving It Instead of Losing It
Provides historical perspective of our body's need
for motion and gives ways to fit movement into your
daily schedule

STEP TEN   87
Practicing Good Posture
Reviews good posture practice and illustrates
specific posture tips for many common activities
and positions

REVIEW...   111

SOME FINAL THOUGHTS   115

Appendix   119
A. Checking and Recording Your Own Posture   120
B. Bookmark/Monitor Placard   126
C. Weekly Self-Care Record Form   127
D. About Gravity   131
E. The Seated Spine   134
F. Injury Prevention   146
G. Winning the Battle with Back Pain   154

Notes Section   170

About the Author   171

Glossary   172

Bibliography   173

Index   174

ILLUSTRATIONS

Subject (# of Graphics)	Page
Good vs. poor working posture (1)	16
Fig. 1: Back view neutral spine (1)	23
Fig. 2: Side view neutral spine (1)	23
Fig. 3: Parts of a spinal segment (2)	24
Fig. 4: The sit bones (1)	25
Fig. 5: Connective soft tissues (1)	28
Fig. 6: Soft tissues / body movement (3)	29
Fig. 7: The process of poor posture (4)	32
Fig. 8: Poor posture and surfaces (1)	33
Fig. 9: Healthy and unhealthy spines (4)	36
Fig. 10: Strain of postural muscles (1)	37
Fig. 11: Feeling the natural spinal arch (1)	41
Fig. 12: Normal lower back arch (2)	42
Fig. 13: Rounded lower back arch (2)	43
Fig. 14: Spinal contours in athletes (3)	45
Fig. 15: The ribcage area (1)	49
Fig. 16: Sitting and head bending (2)	50
Fig. 17: Sitting and arm raising (2)	51
Fig. 18: Sitting and pelvic tilting (2)	52
Fig. 19: Slumping vs. upright sitting (2)	53
Fig. 20: Body position for sitting (2)	55
Fig. 21: Seatback position for sitting (2)	55
Fig. 22: Correct sitting posture (1)	57
Fig. 23: Slumping posture (1)	60
Fig. 24: Poor posture and injury (1)	61
Bookmark/Monitor Placard (1)	62
Self-Care Record (1)	64
Fig. 25: Slumping and rounding (2)	68
Rolled towel for the neck (3)	69
Extension stretching (1)	70

Fig. 26: Taking the stairs (1)   75
60 Second Workout: leg pumps (1)   76
60 Second Workout: leg stretch (1)   76
60 Second Workout: body rotations (2)   77
60 Second Workout: seated sit-ups (2)   77
60 Second Workout: shoulder rolls (1)   78
60 Second Workout: body stretch (1)   78
60 Second Workout: squats (1)   79
60 Second Workout: bun busters (1)   79
Fig. 27: Range of motion stretch (3)   80
Sit disc mobilization chair and disc (1)   82
Sit disc mobilization motions (4)   83
Fig. 28: Hamstrings and pelvic tilting (2)   85
Fig. 29: Stretching the hamstrings (1)   85
Posture tips: proper sitting (2)   90
Posture tips: objects in back pocket (1)   90
Posture tips: driving position (2)   91
Posture tips: reclining (2)   91
Posture tips: reading (2)   92
Posture tips: watching TV (2)   92
Posture tips: reading or TV in bed (2)   93
Posture tips: head-forward effort (1)   93
Posture tips: kids and video games (2)   95
Ergonomics: position for the hands (2)   97
Ergonomics: position for the desktop (2)   97
Ergonomics: desktop arrangement (2)   97
Ergonomics: monitor height (2)   99
Ergonomics: desktop vs. laptop (2)   99
Ergonomics: regular vs. short keyboard (2)   99
Ergonomics: arm motion in mouse use (2)   101
Ergonomics: shoulder/arm position (2)   101
Posture tips: standing and bending (2)   105
Posture tips: stand and walk (2)   105

Posture tips: sleeping on the back (2)   107
Posture tips: sleeping on the side (2)   107
Posture tips: pillow for the legs (2)   107
Posture tips: phone hand vs. headset (2)   109
Posture tips: lifting technique (2)   109
Fig. 30: Checking posture (1)   120
Fig. 31: Poor vs. good front posture (2)   123
Fig. 32: Poor vs. good side posture (2)   125
Monitor Placard Instructions (1)   126
Weekly Self-Care Record Form (1)   130
Poor posture and gravity   133
Parts of a spinal segment (2)   135
Lumbar spine and disc (1)   136
Muscle activity and level arm (4)   138
Slumping posture and the sit bones (1)   140
Reclining posture and the neck (1)   141
Recommended working posture (1)   143
Recommended resting posture (1)   144
Risk factors: lifting charts (4)   149
Risk factors: seated deskwork charts (4)   151
Risk factors: repetitive motions charts (4)   153
Flat back stretch (1)   159
Cat-cow yoga stretch (2)   160
Standing side stretch (2)   161
Knee-to-opposite-shoulder stretch (1)   162
Alternating arm/leg extension exercise (1)   162

PREFACE

In the early years of reality TV, there was a program on the Fox network called *The Swan*. Each episode introduced a small group of female contestants with various unsightly physical features. The idea of the program was to learn about the hardships each contestant had endured due to their cosmetic challenges and then watch them being transformed from Ugly Ducklings to Beautiful Swans over a three month period through various surgeries, makeovers, diets, physical training, and counseling. Each episode ended with a "reveal" where the curtains were drawn back and the contestants took center stage to show off the final results of their intensive transformations. Eventually one contestant from each episode was chosen to move on and compete at the end of the season for title of *The Swan*.

There were many eye-opening transformations during the two seasons the program aired, but one particular observation kept "revealing" itself to me over and over again. Despite the boot camp of specialists—including coaches, therapists, trainers, cosmetic surgeons, and dentists—and all the advanced procedures, makeup, hair styling, and new clothes, the Swans still had Ugly Duckling posture. Why? Because no amount of cosmetic enhancements, muscle hardening, or self-image building had addressed issues specifically relating to the shape of the spine and posture awareness.

Most of the contestants had little poise when they started and no more when they finished, despite any other physical or psychological changes, as judged by their stature when at rest and their gait while in motion. In the absence of structural changes to skeletal alignment, and without the necessary attention to posture, it follows there were no functional improvements in their body positions and movements.

Did anyone else notice? A lot of people probably sensed something was awkward but couldn't put their finger on exactly what it was. Our society today generally has minimal self-awareness of posture, and popular culture even seems to promote a slouchy stance, but there is something subconscious in us that still recognizes good body form when we see it and associates that quality with grace, health, and distinction. The opposites also apply.

For that reason, and because of the rapidly growing worldwide epidemic of preventable posture-related health problems, I have written this new book that encompasses and greatly expands on the content of my earlier work *Sitting Pretty*. The new title, *The Science of Sitting Made Simple*, represents a greater emphasis and integration of information from research on the subject of the seated human body. Get ready to enjoy learning more about posture and what you can do to make yours better than ever—with as little time and effort as possible.

DEAR READER

Every book that offers advice on subjects related to health requires a few extra words of caution (otherwise known as a disclaimer). So let's get through this and then move on to the main course.

The information contained in this book should not be used to self-diagnose or treat any condition and is no substitute for professional healthcare. Always consult with your doctor and discuss your plans before starting, changing or stopping any program that may affect your wellbeing, especially if you are (or should be) under care for any medical condition.

Be sure to proceed with caution when altering any established habits or routines that have the potential to affect your health. The human body can adapt to almost anything, good or bad, given enough time. Just as a diet and exercise program can be beneficial when implemented properly, or harmful when adopted too abruptly, posture improvement practiced safely requires a step-by-step approach. Don't be in too much of a hurry to change something that has probably taken a while to develop—just be consistent.

With consistency, you can use the same physical forces and tissue properties that have been working against you, promoting deformity and degeneration, to work for you, supporting posture restoration.

In reality, time will pass regardless of what you do. Ask yourself, "what can I do now to be better off next year?"

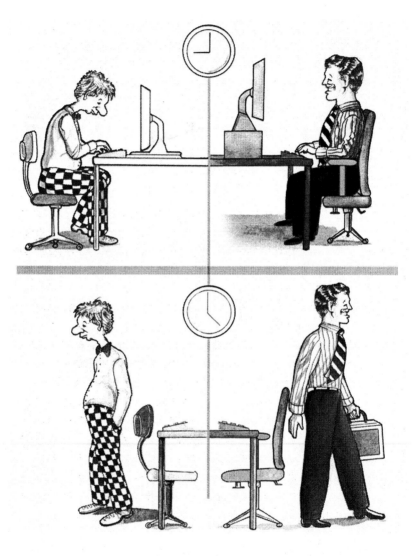

How do you feel at the end of the day?

INTRODUCTION

Most people today spend more time sitting than they do in any other position. We usually sit while we work, commute, eat, and relax; that's a lot of sitting! For something we do so often, most of us aren't very good at it. Unfortunately, many people will eventually experience unnecessary pain, predictable degenerative changes, and even physical impairments and workplace disability as a result of poor posture habits. What we need is a commonsense understanding of why posture is so important that it can literally shape our future, with a commonsense approach for learning how to sit properly. This book aims to do just that, in ten easy steps.

Putting good posture into practice requires that you have the understanding, awareness, and ability to correctly position and move your body. Some people have the physical capacity to place their body in good posture positions but lack the know-how or concern to do so. Others want to enjoy all the benefits that attention to their body's alignment can bring but have become so badly misshapen, or restricted in their flexibility, that they cannot "straighten up." Most people will fit somewhere between those two groups. Whatever category you fall into, help is on the way.

These pages include need-to-know information about the human body that will serve as a foundation for your understanding of the proper posture forms as well as the damaging effects of poor posture. Knowledge is power, so be sure to take whatever time is needed to empower yourself with this important information - after all, no one can improve your own posture except you!

As you read through each step, remember that poor posture habits, like other bad habits, can be changed by replacing old patterns of behavior with new and better ones. Use the notes section in the back of the book to write down to-do items or inspirations that come to you along the way. Although your body and mind may resist change, if you put the practical ideas found in these pages to use gradually, you will succeed, as the long-term rewards far outweigh the short-term effort that is required.

Much of this book concerns the normal shape of the spine and the neutral position that maintains the spine's normal shape. This is called "static posture." Static posture is important because 1) the majority of people these days do spend most of their time in stationary positions and 2) the foundation of body motion comes from stability of the spine and pelvis. Strength and balanced motion of the head, trunk, and extremities cannot be initiated and maintained without the support of a stable central frame. Static posture is about that structure which gives rise to the function of movement. Just as structure and function are intimately related, so too must good posture practice include both proper static position and periodic body mobility, as you will discover.

Once you have finished reviewing all the simple posture awareness, stretch, and movement tips found herein, it is recommended that you start adding these into your routine gradually, perhaps experimenting with one or two of the techniques each day to find which ones work best for you. When you begin to focus on sitting in a better position, try it for only one hour at first. After that, work up to two hours of proper sitting, and so on. After enough time and repetition, good posture will replace poor posture as a habit, as will incorporating quick bouts of motion into the otherwise sedentary existence of deskwork.

For greater depth, details, and insights into the subject of sitting posture, refer to the Appendix sections on "Gravity" and "The Seated Spine" for the current evidence-based research on the seated human body. Information on avoiding trouble before it strikes can be found in the section "Injury Prevention." For people already suffering from the ill-effects of poor posture or back injuries, there is a section called "Winning the Battle with Back Pain." Don't be afraid of any unfamiliar words, as terminology not commonly used in everyday language will be explained.

One final note: Quality is more important than quantity. Busy people want focused, reliable information with self-help techniques that can be practiced in just minutes a day. Therefore, you'll find nothing esoteric, redundant, self-promoting, or overly time-consuming filling the pages of this posture book. Only what you must know about sitting and posture reinforced with dozens of practical illustrations—because a picture really is worth a thousand words. Read on!

For I believe that much of a man's character will be found betoken in his backbone. I would rather feel your spine than your skull, whoever you are. A thin joist of a spine never yet upheld a full and noble soul. I rejoice in my spine, as in the firm audacious staff of that flag which I fling half out to the world.

Melville, *Moby Dick*

Understanding Your Spine's Normal Shape

You should learn:

a. Why the spine has a definite shape
b. What that shape is
c. How the parts of the spine work

STEP ONE
Understanding Your Spine's Normal Shape

Your spine's shape accounts for its ability to be strong and flexible at the same time, which is no easy task for any structure that functions as a central support. As viewed from the back, a healthy spine is straight, like a vertical column (Figure 1). As viewed from the side, a healthy spine has contours (Figure 2). In the neck area (*cervical*), the spine curves toward the front of the body. In the ribcage area (*thoracic*), the spine curves toward the back of the body. In the lower back area (*lumbar*), the spine curves again toward the front of the body. In the pelvic area, the base of the spine (*sacrum*) attaches to the two pelvic bones (*pelvis*). Notice that the spine is not one continuous structure but rather a chain of inter-connecting segments.

The upright position of the spine helps it resist the downward pull of gravity, which is a greater force acting on the body than most people realize. The spine can most efficiently support the body when it is aligned vertically from top to bottom. On the other hand, the spine can best provide flexibility and muscle leverage when it is contoured from front to back. Each contour acts as a pivot point, much like the centerpiece of a seesaw that you might find in a child's playground. Just as a well-balanced seesaw can lift and move with greater ease than an unbalanced one, a spine with well-developed contours is stronger and more flexible than a spine without proper contours.

Because of the important role the structure of your spine plays in both support and movement, your spine is both straight and contoured. A healthy spine must be shaped this way for maximum strength, flexibility, and good posture.

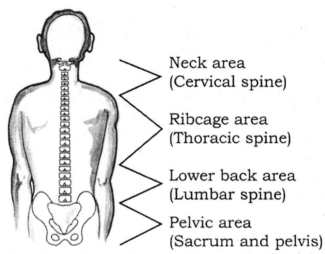

Neck area
(Cervical spine)

Ribcage area
(Thoracic spine)

Lower back area
(Lumbar spine)

Pelvic area
(Sacrum and pelvis)

Figure 1. Back view of the neutral spine: major areas

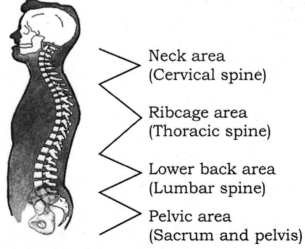

Neck area
(Cervical spine)

Ribcage area
(Thoracic spine)

Lower back area
(Lumbar spine)

Pelvic area
(Sacrum and pelvis)

Figure 2. Side view of the neutral spine: major areas

Let's take a closer look at an individual spine segment, as seen from a side view (Figure 3). Each segment consists of a bone whose proper name is *vertebra* (which is why the entire spine is also known as the vertebral column). The main weight-bearing part at the front of the vertebra is called the *vertebral body*, and behind that are the interconnecting *facet joints* that guide movement of one vertebra on another. Between each vertebra is an *intervertebral disc* that helps to a) distribute weight through the spine, b) create space between each vertebra, and c) hold the vertebrae together. It should be noted that the forward contours of the spine as seen from the side views of the neck and lower back are mainly due to the wedged shape of the intervertebral discs in those areas of the spine.

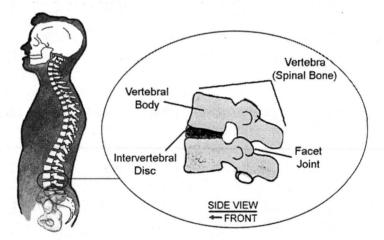

Figure 3. The parts of a spinal segment

The large inverted triangular bone at the base of the spine is the *sacrum* (as seen in Figure's 1 and 2 on the previous page), which is sandwiched between the two pelvic bones that make up the *pelvis*. The bottom of the pelvic bones that you sit on are formally called the *ischial tuberosities* and informally called the "sit bones" (Figure 4).

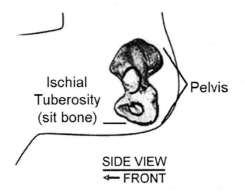

Figure 4. The "sit bones" are at the bottom of the pelvis— one on either side of the body. As you sit, your pelvis can easily rock back and forth on these two bony prominences.

It is interesting to note that the spinal contour in the ribcage area (*thoracic* spine), called the primary curve because it is first to develop, results from our rounded fetal position in the womb. After we are born and gain the ability to hold our head up, a secondary curve develops in the *cervical* spine. With crawling and, later, walking we also develop a secondary curve in the *lumbar* spine. So our primary curve in the mid-back develops inside the womb's near-weightless environment, while our secondary curves in the neck and lower back develop later in response to muscle effort against gravity. It seems we then spend the rest of our lives deforming those secondary spinal contours by returning to a fetal posture, outside of the womb and in a chair.

Count on Your Spine

Most of us are born with thirty-three vertebrae in our spines. The four lowest vertebrae eventually join together to form the coccyx (tailbone), and the next five vertebrae join together to form the sacrum (spinal base). The fusion of these lower spinal bones into the coccyx and the sacrum is usually completed by age thirty. Moving up the spine, there are five lumbar vertebrae in the lower back, twelve thoracic vertebrae in the mid-back (which connect to twelve pairs of ribs), and seven vertebrae in the neck. So, at full maturity, we normally have twenty-four freely moving vertebrae in our spines. Less than ten percent of the time, people are born with an extra lumbar vertebra; therefore, they will have twenty-five vertebrae in their spines at adulthood.

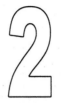

Keeping It Together

You should learn:

a. What holds the spine together
b. How the spine can move freely yet maintain its normal shape

STEP TWO
Keeping It Together

The spine is a stack of loosely fitting vertebrae that are held together by *connective soft tissue* structures made of muscles, tendons, ligaments, fasciae (thin tough wrapping), and discs. These connective soft tissues run the entire length of the spine and help maintain its overall shape. Think of the spinal bones (vertebrae) as giving rigid support to the spine, and the connective soft tissues as giving flexible support to the spine.

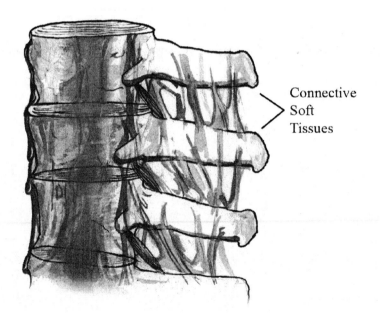

Connective
Soft
Tissues

Figure 5. The soft tissues connecting the vertebrae from top to bottom play a major role in the position and movement of the spine.

It is a normal function of the spine to temporarily change in shape when accommodating shifts in body posture during physical activity and rest. Varying degrees of stretch in your connective soft tissues make this possible and assist your spine in "remembering" its normal shape again when you move your body back to a neutral position. In other words, it is the connective soft tissues and not the vertebrae themselves that are primarily responsible for your spine's mobility.

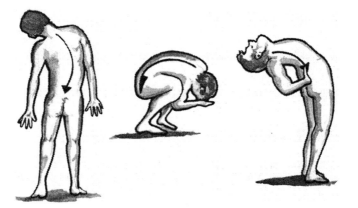

Figure 6. The flexible soft tissues of the spine work together to allow body movement; their elasticity guides the spine back to its normal shape each time you return to a neutral position.

You're Well Connected

A joint is the point at which two bones are connected. A ligament connects bone to bone and helps to hold a joint together. A tendon connects muscle to bone, and the action of a muscle moves a joint. Muscles are fairly elastic and tend to bounce back to their resting shape after contracting or stretching. Ligaments are not very flexible and have a slow, creep-like quality that does not favor the return of a stretched ligament back to its original shape. Tendons are rather stiff, like coiled springs, with minimal stretchability, increasing rebound energy as they lengthen, and an overall tendency to retain their shape.

Learning How You Get Bent out of Shape

You should learn:

a. How poor posture changes the shape of your spine
b. Why it can become difficult to straighten up

STEP THREE
Learning How You Get Bent out of Shape

Poor posture is usually a bad habit that develops and persists over many years. When you hold any body position for long periods of time, your spine is gradually reshaped into that very position through an adaptation of the connective soft tissues. These connective soft tissues that keep your spine in place eventually lose their ability to guide your spine back to its normal shape under the repeated strain of poor posture. It is for this reason that your spine tends to become shaped exactly like the position you're most often in.

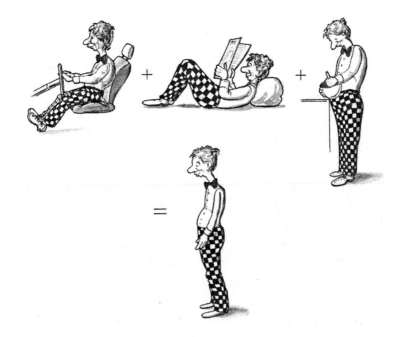

Figure 7. The process that results in poor posture

The process that results in poor posture involves placing your body in the same incorrect position, even with different activities. You get bent out of shape by sitting, lying, and standing in a way that repeatedly stresses your spine in a similar pattern. Over time, the connective soft tissues surrounding your spine become overly slack or increasingly rigid, causing a progressive change from your normal alignment.

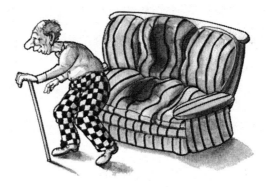

Figure 8. Beware of poor posture and the sitting and sleeping surfaces that contribute to it!

If you mold your spine into an abnormal shape, changing from healthy posture to poor posture, eventually you lose the ability to freely return to an upright position. That's why it's important that the sitting and sleeping surfaces you rest on most often are contoured to you, not the other way around, or you may end up shaped just like that old couch. Poor posture habits are a big part of the progressive deformity of the body's frame in older people.

The Modern-Day Hunchbacks

The word dowager refers to an older, wealthy woman. A "dowager's hump" refers to a rounded deformity of the upper back also known as hyperkyphosis. The relation between older women and that hump in the upper back has to do with osteoporosis. In advanced osteoporosis, the spinal bones can become brittle and cave in at the front edges of the vertebrae. This creates wedge-shaped vertebrae that severely round the upper back. Can men, younger women, and even children or teenagers develop a "dowager's hump?" The answer is yes, and it has nothing at all to do with osteoporosis. Postural kyphosis is the most common cause of excess rounding of the upper back and is completely attributable to poor posture habits like slumping.

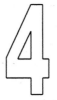

Understanding How Degeneration Happens

You should learn:

a. Why the spine and soft tissues degenerate
b. What the symptoms of degeneration are
c. How to avoid the degenerative process

STEP FOUR
Understanding How Degeneration Happens

With proper posture, the normal shape of the spine is maintained, and weight that is carried on the vertebrae and connective soft tissues is shared evenly. With poor posture, the spine is bent from its normal shape. Strain on the vertebrae and soft tissues becomes focused on one section more than another. A spinal section under greater strain will respond by gradually hardening against the added pressure. Extra bone deposits harden vertebrae, while scar tissue deposits harden the connective soft tissues.

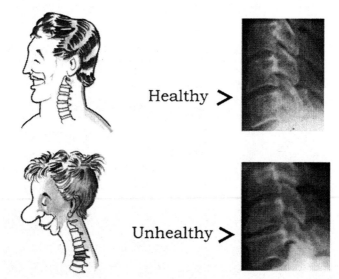

Healthy >

Unhealthy >

Figure 9. Examples of a healthy (top image) and an unhealthy (bottom image) shape in the neck area of the spine. In the unhealthy spine, the vertebrae are under greater strain, leading to deterioration of the discs and extra bone deposits in the vertebrae.

The end result of hardening is degeneration, in which the vertebrae become thicker and form jagged edges, the discs between the vertebrae become brittle and thin, and the soft tissues become rigid. Degeneration typically causes joints to feel stiff and muscles to feel weak and tight. Normal mobility may be lost.

Good posture practice helps avoid degeneration by maintaining the normal shape of the spine to equally share the compressing force of gravity. Also, regular stretching or activity breaks during long sitting periods helps to stimulate blood flow and nourish postural muscles that need more incoming oxygen and outgoing metabolic waste products.

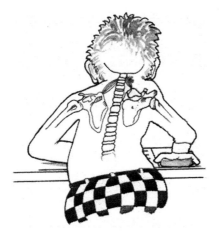

Figure 10. Unhealthy posture and inactivity strain postural muscles and slow circulation in the body, leading to scar tissue deposits. Muscles that are held in an isometric (static/same length) contraction, as postural muscles often are, need only be tensed at 40% of their maximum effort to restrict blood flow.

We Are All Scarred for Life

Scar tissue is a natural result of the healing process. When any kind of damage occurs, the body has only a limited ability to restore injured tissue back to pre-damaged condition. Therefore, scar tissue will be used as a filler to replace nonrepairable tissue. Scar tissue is a fibrous, dense, less functional, and inferior-quality replacement of healthy tissue. That explains why a person can never truly recover 100% after an injury, and also why older people tend to have more health problems (they've been around longer to accumulate more damage). When injury happens (from acute trauma, repetitive motions, postural strain, and so on), it isn't a question of whether or not scar tissue will be laid down, but rather how extensive and how well-adapted the remaining scar will be. In most cases, a focus on body symmetry, balanced forces, and frequent mobility are the key factors that will help resolve an injury as rapidly and completely as possible.

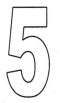

Understanding Your Correct Posture

You should learn:

a. How to find the forward arch in your lower back with your spine in a neutral position
b. What proper and improper sitting does to your lower back arch
c. Who uses their well-developed spinal contours to win

STEP FIVE
Understanding Your Correct Posture

Good posture involves maintaining the normal shape of the spine. When sitting, it is especially important to maintain the natural forward arch in your lower back (*lumbar lordosis*). To test for the arch in your lumbar area, try the following:

a. From a standing position, slowly back up (don't lean) against a wall until your head, shoulder blades, and buttocks touch the wall. Having your head, ribcage and pelvis aligned in this neutral position brings your spine toward its normal shape. (If you have forward head carriage, very rounded shoulders, or a protruding buttocks, you may find it difficult to vertically align yourself in this position.)

b. Place one hand behind you, between your lower back and the wall, just above where your beltline would be. If you have the correct arch in the lumbar spine, your hand will slide into the space just above your pelvis and below your shoulder blades (Figure 11). Try to get an idea of about how deep and tall the space is relative to the size of your hand.

This shows you that when you are in an upright position, the normal shape of your lumbar spine has a forward arch, or lordosis, that must be supported when you are sitting correctly. If this lumbar arch, or lordosis, is not supported when you are sitting, your lower spine will flatten or round out of its normal and healthy shape, with undesirable consequences throughout your body.

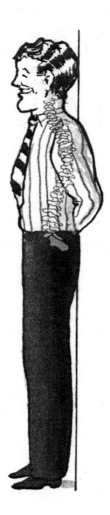

Figure 11: Feeling your natural spinal arch in the lower back (lumbar lordosis)

As you already know from Step Three, posture habits can affect the shape of the spine. Good posture supports the spine's normal contours while poor posture deforms them. In the proper sitting position, the top of the pelvis is slightly tilted forward to maintain the natural lumbar lordosis, disc shape, and facet joint positions in the lower back, all of which helps to distribute the upper body weight evenly through the spine (Figure 12). Maintaining the normal contours of the spine, angle of the disc, and spacing of the facet joints provides the structural reinforcement needed for proper strength and stability.

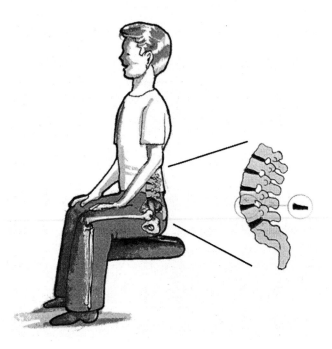

Figure 12. Maintaining the arch in the lower back (lumbar lordosis) facilitates normal weight distribution and disc shape in the spine.

Improper sitting causes the pelvis to tilt backward, resulting in a loss of the natural forward arch in the lower back (Figure 13). Without the lumbar lordosis, the back rounds outward, shifting the body's weight distribution forward and causing compression and flattening of the discs as well as altered weight-bearing of the lumbar facet joints.

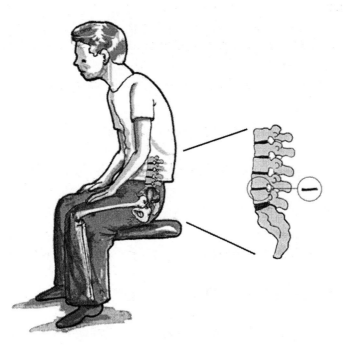

Figure 13. Rounding the lower back shifts weight forward on the spine and flattens the disc.

That is why proper sitting and lifting techniques always include attention to maintaining the normal shape of the spine, including the forward arch of the lower back, creating a solid foundation of support with proper weight distribution.

People who participate in sports, using their bodies for activities requiring strength and stability, usually have well-developed spinal contours, including the lumbar arch, or lordosis. To stay competitive in professional sports, athletes need excellent form to maximize their potential for performance. Therefore, you will often notice a healthy forward arch in the lower back of any great athlete, present both at rest and during participation in their sport (Figure 14), providing a natural edge above competitors who lack the normal spinal contour.

Remember that in Step One, "Understanding Your Spine's Normal Shape," you learned the contours of the spine, including the lumbar lordosis, are present to give greater strength and flexibility. If you have a well-developed arch in your lower spine, your back is much stronger than it would be without one. However, because the lower spine is normally contoured forward and not flat, it does requires special attention and accommodation when sitting—as you will learn in the next step.

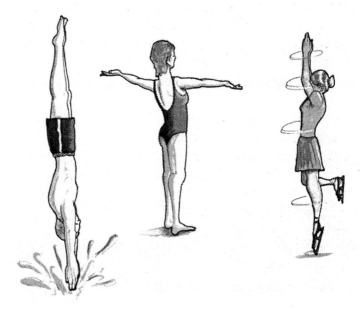

Figure 14. The contours of the spine give added strength and stability that are easily recognizable in the graceful form of athletes.

What's Normal?

Most people age 30 and above will have some "normal" degree of breakdown in the discs of their lower spine, a process called degenerative disc disease. One main feature of the degenerative process is dehydration and shrinkage of the discs. There are different theories as to why the discs dry out, but it is well known that the constant movement of fluids in and out of the discs is needed to bring in nutrients and allow the discs to stay healthy. Consider that sitting forward in your chair with your back rounded creates almost twice as much pressure inside the discs of your lower back compared to sitting erect (which has an effect on the discs similar to wringing out a sponge). When poor sitting posture, which raises disc pressure, is combined with prolonged periods of sitting where there is not much movement of fluids in and out of the discs, degenerative disc disease would seem to be a likely consequence—and maybe better described as average rather than normal.

Sitting up When You Sit Down

You should learn:

a. What part of your body to focus on when sitting up
b. Why your body becomes impaired if you slump
c. How to put yourself and your chair into the correct position for sitting

STEP SIX
Sitting up When You Sit Down

Proper sitting is all about the position of the middle part of your body (the ribcage area) because your head, your arms, and your lower spine all attach to your ribcage. Changes in the position of your ribcage affect the forward pitch of your head, the height of your arms, and the arch of your lower back (lordosis).

Often people get tired and frustrated trying to force their "head up and shoulders back" because they are letting their back slump at the same time. Attempting to focus your attention on keeping your head up and your shoulders back while you sit with a sunken chest and collapsed ribcage is fighting a losing battle—especially if you have work to concentrate on or you just want to relax.

Why struggle trying to maintain good sitting posture by constantly tracking where your head, arms, and lower back are positioned if doing so is impractical and distracting? It is much easier to sit with a healthy and youthful upright posture by simply remembering the one big part in the middle of your body, your ribcage area. (The ribcage is made of twelve matching pairs of ribs that attach to the thoracic spine. The neck, or cervical spine, attaches to the thoracic spine at the top. The shoulder blades, or scapulae, are positioned over the sides of the ribcage. The lower back, or lumbar spine, attaches to the thoracic spine at the bottom—all as shown in Figure 15.)

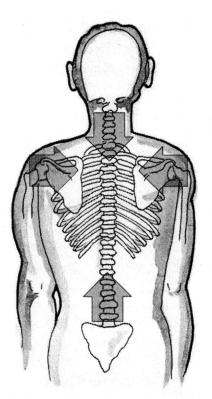

Figure 15. Your head, arms, and lower back attach to the ribcage area of your thoracic spine.

To understand the connection between your ribcage and the position and movement of your head, arms and lower back, try the following experiments. You will need to alternate between a slumping and an upright sitting position to feel the effects that changing posture has on head posture, shoulder and arm movement, and the lower back arch, as follows:

Head Posture

a. Sit near the edge of a chair.

b. Slump so that your back becomes rounded. Remain in a slumped position and allow your head to slowly bend forward so that your chin comes closer to your chest (a).

c. Next, return your head to an upright position and sit up tall in the chair. Allow your head to slowly bend forward again (b). You will notice that it is not so easy to drop your head forward while sitting up straight.

This demonstrates that upright sitting helps you maintain proper head position in your body's mid-line, which is important to preventing unhealthy and disfiguring forward head posture.

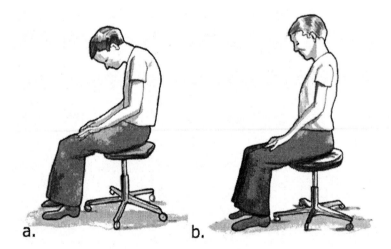

a.   b.

Figure 16. The upright sitting position makes it easier to avoid excessive forward head bending.

Shoulder and Arm Movement

a. Slump again so that your back becomes rounded a second time.

b. Remain in a slumped position and slowly raise your arm up overhead (a).

c. Next, lower your arm, then sit up tall and slowly raise your arm overhead again. You will notice that it is easier to raise your arm higher while sitting up straight (b).

This demonstrates that upright sitting helps you maintain the normal mobility of your arms, which is important when you use a keyboard or mouse.

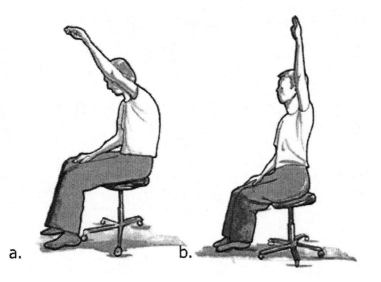

a.   b.

Figure 17. The upright sitting position makes it easier to freely move your shoulders and arms.

Lower Back Arch

a. Slump again so that your back becomes rounded once more.

b. Remain in a slumped position and place your hands on your sides at waist level. Your hands should be resting on top of your pelvic bone with your fingers facing forward and slightly upward, and your thumbs facing backward and slightly downward (a).

c. Now slowly sit upright and tall and allow your hands to rotate with your pelvic bone as you move into upright posture. You will notice that, as you transition from slumping to sitting upright, your fingers roll downward while your thumbs roll upward (b).

This demonstrates that upright sitting allows the proper forward pelvic tilt, which is important to maintaining the arch in your lower back.

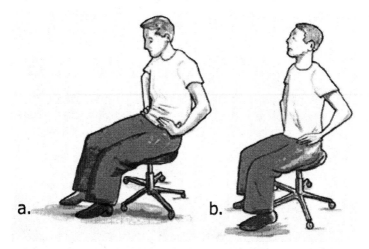

Figure 18. The upright sitting position makes it easier to maintain the proper arch in your lower back.

The previous experiments helped you experience that in the common poor posture habit of dropping your ribcage down (slumping), your head is bent forward and your pelvis tilts backward, which flattens out the natural forward arch of your lower back (a). In the correct sitting posture (b), your ribcage is held in an upright position, maintaining your lower back arch and pelvic tilt, and allowing your head to more easily stay centered atop your shoulders (Figure 19).

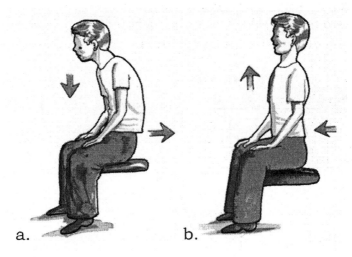

a.   b.

Figure 19.

A. Slumping rounds your back, drops your ribcage, pokes your head forward, and shortens your sitting height.

B. Correct posture keeps your lower back arched, your ribcage elevated, your head aligned, and your body upright.

Another important distinction to be aware of between an upright and a slumping posture is the compression effect on your internal organs. The heart, lungs, and digestive organs all have more room within the body spaces of the thorax and abdomen when you sit in the correct posture. Internal space is important to ensure good circulation, which provides oxygenation, nutrition, and the removal of waste products. If you wish to experience the compression effect of slumping on your internal organs, simply position yourself in posture A from Figure 19 on the previous page and take in a long, deep breath and then slowly exhale. Next, position yourself in posture B and repeat the breathing exercise. You should notice that you were able to breathe in much more deeply and with much less effort in posture B compared to posture A because there is more space for your lungs to expand when you sit in an upright posture.

The instructions that follow will help you better understand the corrections in body position, seat-back position, and lumbar support that often need to be made to help you sit up when you are sitting down. (For information on adapting your sitting position to your workstation, refer to the Step By Step Ergonomic Tune-Up in Step Ten.) Although maintaining good posture may sometimes seem complex or difficult, especially at busy times, all you need to remember is the middle part of your body. Therefore, sitting correctly means simply keeping your ribcage area upright. You can keep your ribcage upright by following a., b., and c.:

a. Correct your body position. Sit as far back into your seat as you can. Your buttocks should be snug against the seatback of your chair. Your feet should be flat on the floor or on a footrest.

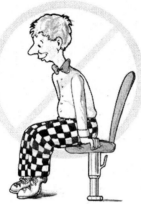
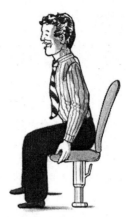

Figure 20.
Incorrect body position
at the edge of the chair
the feet hanging

Correct body position
against the seatback with
with the feet flat

b. Correct your seatback position. Set your
seatback to an upright (nearly vertical) position
that is locked into place so that you can lean
back into your chair without having the seatback
give way.

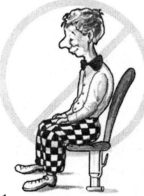
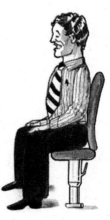

Figure 21.
Incorrect seatback position
results in slumping and
fatigue.

Correct seatback
position is supportive
and relaxing.

After following a. and b., your buttocks and shoulder blades should be touching the seatback of your chair. Your head should be aligned directly above your shoulders. You may feel more upright in your seat than you are used to. Recall that in the previous section, "Understanding Your Correct Posture," your head, ribcage, and pelvis were vertically aligned when you tried the neutral standing position. Although sitting upright and against your seatback may be different from how you used to sit, it is relaxing to allow your upper body weight to rest fully against your seatback. The only remaining instruction is to fill that natural space in the lumbar area of your spine.

c. Insert a lumbar support between the forward curve of your lower back (located just above your belt line) and the seatback. This lumbar support may be a preformed cushion or simply a rolled towel that's just big enough to fill the space between the arch of your lower back and the back of your seat. Whatever you use, make sure it's the proper size so it doesn't push your buttocks and shoulder blades away from the seatback. A lumbar support strip large enough to fill the space of your lumbar arch, but small enough to allow full contact of your sacral/pelvic and thoracic spine regions against your chair, is ideal. Once you have your lumbar support in the correct position, attach it to your seatback. Your back should plug right into your seatback like a matching puzzle piece. Then, just relax your upper body weight into your chair. This is how to achieve an upright, yet fully relaxed, sitting posture.

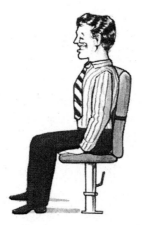

Figure 22. Correct sitting posture with lumbar area support to fill the natural forward arch (lordosis) of the lower back

The key to upright and relaxed sitting is the correct seatback position, proper placement and size of the lumbar support, and the upper body weight resting against the seatback—all of which maximizes weight distribution. If your entire weight rests on one small area of your body, that spot becomes tired and sore very quickly. When your weight is spread out over many areas of your body, less pressure is concentrated on any one spot. That is why sitting with your lower back, your buttocks, and your thighs well supported, and with your feet flat on the floor or footrest, allows you to lean back into your chair and stay upright while remaining relaxed. Check out section E in the Appendix for more information.

Stop Sitting for a Living

The average person living in an industrialized nation and working at a desk job typically spends twelve or more hours per day sitting. This takes into account commute time, work time, meal time, and relaxation time over the course of a day. During those twelve or more hours of sitting, the average-sized person is only burning about 80 calories per hour. Simply standing up will burn 20% more calories, and adding light activity around the office or home while standing will increase energy expenditure 300% over just sitting. With some 25% of English-speaking populations in the world now meeting the definition of obesity, it seems like a good idea to discourage prolonged sitting as a daily routine.

Using Your Awareness to Stop Slumping

You should learn:

a. Why people tend to slump when they sit

b. How slumping can hurt more than just your spine

c. What you can do to boost your posture awareness

STEP SEVEN
Using Your Awareness to Stop Slumping

Most people slump when they sit because they have limited awareness of their bad habit of slumping, or they mistake slumping for relaxation. The truth is, slumping causes fatigue. Just thinking about how you are sitting from time to time will give you the opportunity to greatly improve your posture habits and increase your energy.

Another reason poor posture is so epidemic is that our chairs (as commonly used without added supports) often encourage slumping. This applies to seats in airplanes, theaters, buses, and subways, as well as park benches, couches, and easy chairs. Slumping in your seat may feel relaxing, but it only shifts strain from one part of your body to another.

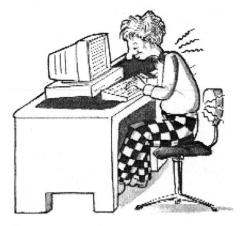

Figure 23. Slumping leads to poor posture, tiredness, and pain.

Slumping is ultimately more tiring than sitting in an upright neutral posture. Slumping is also unattractive and can lead to permanent deformity and degeneration of your spine. Real relaxation comes from keeping your spine in the most balanced and supported position for its natural contours, and from moving to other balanced and supported positions at regular intervals.

Changes in the shape of your spine that accompany slumping also disturb the normal position and coordinated function of your arms and legs. Improper joint alignment and muscular imbalance makes damage from repetitive tasks or athletic activities much more likely, which is *another* good reason to increase your posture awareness.

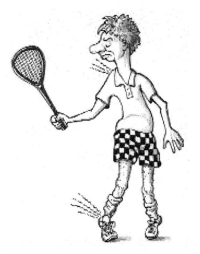

Figure 24. Poor posture increases the likelihood of injury anywhere in your body.

Increasing your posture awareness is a worthwhile goal that can be made easier with several simple suggestions. First, keep in mind that no one is perfect. You will repeatedly forget, remember, and again forget to be aware of your posture. It is better to catch yourself slumping than to slump and never recognize the problem. If you persist in reminding yourself about good posture many times over, eventually you will replace poor posture habits with better ones. It's never too late to start; just be patient with yourself because you are setting out to change a pattern of behavior that has probably been with you for a very long time.

Here are some hints to help you increase your posture awareness:

1. Use visual reminders.

This book comes with a bookmark/monitor placard that can be detached from the back cover and taped to your computer or another convenient place. The placard illustrates poor posture and good posture examples as they relate to desktop layout, workstation setup, and overall body posture. Glancing at the illustrations periodically will help refresh the idea of good posture in your mind throughout the day. You may also choose

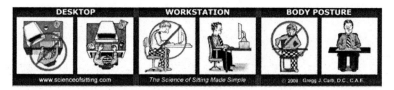

Use of the monitor placard is described in Appendix B.

to post small notes in strategic places (such as the printer or telephone), reminding you to "sit up one inch taller" or "take a short break now."

2. Use ergonomic devices.

Ergonomics is a Greek word first used in the 1800s that literally translates to *work law*. Besides today's popular use of "ergonomics" as a marketing buzzword, in practical terms it really means the interaction between the human body, the tasks performed, and the equipment used. Importantly, the human-body component of that interaction also includes psychological factors that influence much of our behavior.

In fact, it has been shown that the vast majority of workplace injuries are caused by unsafe acts as compared to unsafe conditions. That means most injuries are a result of improper technique or use, poor posture habits, repetitive motions, and a lack of required rest or generalized mobility, as opposed to equipment failure, bad design, and hazardous exposures. In other words, a huge percentage of workplace injuries are completely within the control of the individual worker and his or her choices, awareness, and tendencies. It is for this reason that ergonomic devices alone do not always change poor posture habits.

That being said, the more help you have in the practice of good posture, the easier it will be, and the more likely you are to stick to it and improve. While it is still quite possible to slump in a $1000 ergonomic chair, it is much easier to sit correctly in a chair that is fully supportive and properly adjusted once you completely understand what good posture is and why. Consider other devices such as a footrest, keyboard tray, document holder, laptop holder, telephone headset, and monitor riser to facilitate good form and help you remain mindful of your posture as you work.

3. Use the Self-Care Record form.

Anything worth doing well is worth tracking. Daily use of the Self-Care Record requires only that you check a box after performing any stretch, movement, or breathing exercise. During the few moments throughout your day that it takes to mark the form, you will refresh your awareness about proper body position and regular activity, naturally leading you to better posture.

Weekly Self-Care Record

Date Month/Day	Neck/back Extension Stretch	Stairs or Brisk Walking	Sixty Second Workout	Standing ROM or Sit Disc	Hamstring Stretching	Deep Breathing	Workload	Stress Level	Symptom Status	Comments
Monday	10-15 min. ❏	❏ AM ❏ Noon ❏ PM	❏ AM ❏ Noon ❏ PM	❏ AM ❏ Noon ❏ PM	❏ AM ❏ Noon ❏ PM	❏ AM ❏ Noon ❏ PM	❏ Light ❏ Moderate ❏ Heavy	❏ Low ❏ Med ❏ High	❏ Same ❏ Better ❏ Worse	
Tuesday	10-15 min. ❏	❏ AM ❏ Noon ❏ PM	❏ AM ❏ Noon ❏ PM	❏ AM ❏ Noon ❏ PM	❏ AM ❏ Noon ❏ PM	❏ AM ❏ Noon ❏ PM	❏ Light ❏ Moderate ❏ Heavy	❏ Low ❏ Med ❏ High	❏ Same ❏ Better ❏ Worse	
Wednesday	10-15 min. ❏	❏ AM ❏ Noon ❏ PM	❏ AM ❏ Noon ❏ PM	❏ AM ❏ Noon ❏ PM	❏ AM ❏ Noon ❏ PM	❏ AM ❏ Noon ❏ PM	❏ Light ❏ Moderate ❏ Heavy	❏ Low ❏ Med ❏ High	❏ Same ❏ Better ❏ Worse	
Thursday	10-15 min. ❏	❏ AM ❏ Noon ❏ PM	❏ AM ❏ Noon ❏ PM	❏ AM ❏ Noon ❏ PM	❏ AM ❏ Noon ❏ PM	❏ AM ❏ Noon ❏ PM	❏ Light ❏ Moderate ❏ Heavy	❏ Low ❏ Med ❏ High	❏ Same ❏ Better ❏ Worse	
Friday	10-15 min. ❏	❏ AM ❏ Noon ❏ PM	❏ AM ❏ Noon ❏ PM	❏ AM ❏ Noon ❏ PM	❏ AM ❏ Noon ❏ PM	❏ AM ❏ Noon ❏ PM	❏ Light ❏ Moderate ❏ Heavy	❏ Low ❏ Med ❏ High	❏ Same ❏ Better ❏ Worse	
Saturday	10-15 min. ❏	❏ AM ❏ Noon ❏ PM	❏ AM ❏ Noon ❏ PM	❏ AM ❏ Noon ❏ PM	❏ AM ❏ Noon ❏ PM	❏ AM ❏ Noon ❏ PM	❏ Light ❏ Moderate ❏ Heavy	❏ Low ❏ Med ❏ High	❏ Same ❏ Better ❏ Worse	
Sunday	10-15 min. ❏	❏ AM ❏ Noon ❏ PM	❏ AM ❏ Noon ❏ PM	❏ AM ❏ Noon ❏ PM	❏ AM ❏ Noon ❏ PM	❏ AM ❏ Noon ❏ PM	❏ Light ❏ Moderate ❏ Heavy	❏ Low ❏ Med ❏ High	❏ Same ❏ Better ❏ Worse	

Use of the Self-Care Record is described in Section C of the Appendix.

4. Set a timer.

Hours seem to pass quickly when you are busy. As you become increasingly focused on work, you may temporarily lose awareness of your own needs. If you ignore your body when it whispers about that gradual stiffening of your neck, that growing urge to go to the bathroom, or that slowly but steadily sinking posture, eventually the symptoms will become so deafening you won't be able to pay attention to anything except your body's needs. Instead of waiting for pain to remind you, set your screen saver, your electronic calendar, or a simple wind-up timer to ring every 30—60 minutes, reminding you to adjust your posture, perform a quick stretch or brief exercise, or take a few deep breaths.

5. Notice others.

At this point you have learned a lot about the normal shape of the spine, the soft tissues that hold the spine together, poor posture that bends the spine out of shape, the process of wear and tear in a spine bent out of shape, and the neutral position that aligns your body and maintains the natural forward arch in your lower back. This greater understanding of posture will enable you to notice others around you with a discriminating eye. Poor posture is epidemic in our society and you will see glaring postural faults everywhere— heads jutted forward, shoulders rolled inward, upper backs hunched over, lower backs rounded out, sunken chests, etc. Use those examples as a reminder of what *not* to do to avoid looking inches shorter and years older than you really are.

The Best Chair for You

As much time as we spend sitting, a good chair is a wise investment in the same way that a good mattress can help improve your sleep. (And considering that time in bed and time in an office chair probably make up a significant portion of your adult life, these are not the items to skimp on) The best definition of a good chair would be one that makes you forget it is even there. Because body types are so different, some chairs will fit more naturally than others. Of course, the more adjustable a chair is, the more likely you are to find the correct settings for your particular shape. The message here is that you need to try the chair on for size just like you would a pair of shoes. Chairs these days come with a surprising selection of optional equipment, so do some homework before buying more or less chair than you really need. Top-quality, modern office chairs can cost from several hundred to over a thousand dollars. A few big names in the office furniture industry are Humanscale, Herman Miller, and Steelcase. For further information, search the Internet for "office chair ratings" or similar wording—and no matter what chair you end up with, always practice good sitting posture!

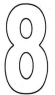

Undoing Damage with Extension Stretching

You should learn:

a. How improper sitting rounds your body
b. What you can do to stretch yourself back into shape

STEP EIGHT
Undoing Damage with Extension Stretching

Recall that chronic slumping looks unattractive and causes injury to the body. Improper sitting also tends to produce the following increasingly painful and disfiguring postural problems:

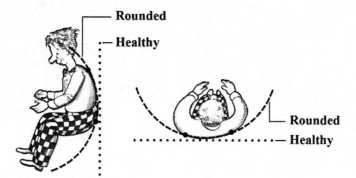

Figure 25. Slumping causes the body to become rounded forward, bending the spine out of its healthy shape from top to bottom and from side to side.

Sitting with good posture helps return the spine and body to an upright position. Additionally, regularly extending *beyond* neutral posture will help you stretch tight muscles (and other connective soft tissues) to regain their natural flexibility and length. The goal is simply to reverse the typical components of poor posture and stretch in that reversed position. In effect, slumping posture is a form of traction (sustained pulling), which stretches your body into forward flexion. To undo that process, you must stretch your body the opposite way into extension and traction yourself in that position.

Ten to fifteen continuous minutes of the following extension stretch, once per day, will help you off-set some of the stress and strain you are likely to accumulate daily when sitting. This is a time-dependent process that cannot be rushed.

If you have hypertension, vascular problems, advanced joint degeneration, cervical disc disease, or any special health concerns, consult your doctor before performing this extension stretch.

Perform your home extension stretch for 10—15 minutes each day, as follows:

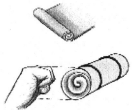

a. Roll a small towel very tightly, so it is about the size of your closed fist (You may wish to place a small wooden dowel or pair of chopsticks in the center to form a more solid core). Place a rubber band on each side of the roll to keep it in place.

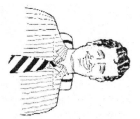

b. Lie on a bed (on your back) with your head near the foot or the side of the bed and place the rolled towel behind the base of your neck.

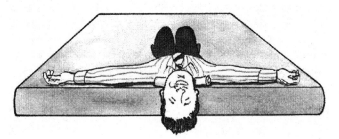

c. Scoot toward the edge of the bed until the rolled towel is near that edge and your head is slightly extended beyond the bed's edge. Keep your head and neck in line with the midline of your body. Don't tilt or turn to one side.

Note: If you feel discomfort when you extend your head, start your first few sessions with your head flat on the bed and gradually extend it over the edge only when you can do so without discomfort.

d. Place your arms straight out (at shoulder level), near the bed's edge. Face the palms of your hands upward.

Note: If you feel discomfort when you stretch out your arms, start your first few sessions with your arms by your side and gradually bring them out to shoulder level only when you can do so without discomfort.

e. Bend your knees and place your feet flat on the bed. Keep your knees apart (about as wide as your hips). You may use a pillow under your knees for comfort.

After 10—15 minutes, gradually slide your body up and lie in a neutral position on top of your bed (with your head and neck fully supported on the bed) and rest a few moments before rising.

Don't Get Ahead of Yourself

Almost everyone wants to get ahead of where they are now, which is fine so long as that phrase remains a figure of speech and does not become a physical reality. The common posture deformity in which the head and neck jut forward in relation to the rest of the body is called Forward Head Posture. The condition is a predictable result of sitting, standing, and/or lying with the head displaced forward of the shoulders for prolonged periods of time, which is what happens with slumping in a chair, standing or walking with a sunken chest, or sleeping on the back with a big pillow under the head. Forward Head Posture has been linked to degenerative spinal changes, muscle tension, impaired breathing capacity, jaw pain, headaches, stiff neck, and even increased mortality among older people. Fixing the problem requires stretches, exercises, and, most importantly, corrected posture practices. Professional treatment and guidance should be considered. As always, though, an ounce of prevention is worth a pound of cure. In the effort to get ahead, which often requires a lot of extra deskwork, remember to keep your head on straight!

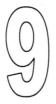

Moving It Instead of Losing It

You should learn:

a. Why inactivity is harmful to your body
b. How to add mobility into your daily routine
c. What leg muscles in sitters need special attention

STEP NINE
Moving It Instead of Losing It

The human body has many bones, joints, and muscles because we are made for motion. From a historical perspective, until very recently we had to be active to survive. Work, play, everyday chores, and getting from place to place all meant constant physical activity. As a consequence of the automation of many tasks, we can now work and play without moving much more than our fingertips. Our routine chores and commuting often involve no more than sitting and waiting.

The workings of our body were not designed for this inactivity. Lack of motion decreases blood circulation, respiration, and fluid exchange. This reduced blood flow and decreased oxygen to already misused and understretched muscles is a major factor in repetitive strain injuries. The solution is motion.

Even if you have perfect posture, you need periodic bouts of mobility to keep you alert and to keep your body flexible. Move your body in a way that is intense enough to increase your heart and lung activity (such as climbing a few flights of stairs or walking briskly) in five-minute increments at least three times each day (mid-morning, lunch, mid-afternoon). That's only 3% of an eight-hour shift, which is a small investment of time that pays big returns of greater energy and productivity—meaning you ultimately get more done in less time. Also, as a general rule, try to avoid sitting still continuously for more than half an hour.

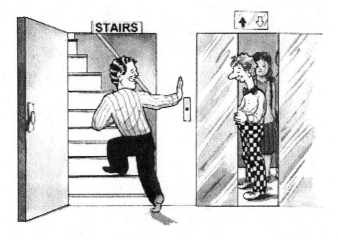

Figure 26. Move your body by taking the stairs!

A quick and easy way to get some motion into your day, one minute at a time, is by performing one or more of the following mobility practices. You don't even have to leave your desk!:

• The Sixty Second Workout (pages 76—79)
• A simple range of motion stretch (page 80)
• Taking a deep breath (page 81)
• Using the "sit disc" (pages 82—83)

Another important mobility issue for people that sit a lot concerns flexibility of the muscles in the back of the thighs (the hamstrings). Tight hamstring muscles can be a cause or a result of poor posture and can create problems with sitting, standing, walking, running, or climbing. Special attention to the hamstrings can help both seated and standing postures:

• Get a leg up (pages 84—85)

Sixty Second Workout

Perform the following Sixty Second Workout, in whole or in part, throughout your day for greater energy and flexibility.

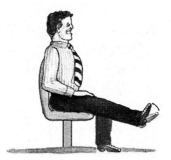

1. Leg Pumps

Duration: Ten seconds. Begin by sitting tall and supported by your seat back. Raise your right leg parallel to the floor. Flex, then point, your right foot. Repeat the flexing and pointing five times, then lower your leg. Repeat with your left leg.

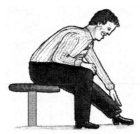

2. Leg Stretch

Duration: Ten seconds. Begin by sitting on the edge of your chair. Extend your right leg while keeping your right foot on the floor. Slowly reach your right arm toward your right foot then gently hold for five seconds. Return to an upright position and repeat using your left leg and left arm (as shown).

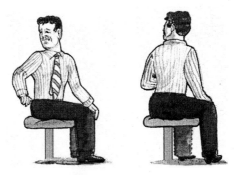

3. Torso and Head Rotation

Duration: Ten seconds. Begin by sitting tall. Keep your legs facing forward. Starting with your lower torso, gently begin to turn your body to your right, continue turning to the right with your chest and shoulders, then with your neck and head. Hold for five seconds. Slowly return to center. Repeat to your left side.

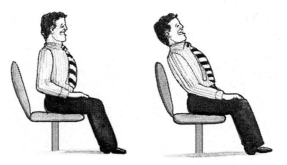

4. Seated Sit-Ups

Duration: Five seconds. Begin by sitting tall on the edge of your chair. Keeping your head and neck in line with your upper back, slowly lean back while keeping an arch in your lower back and keeping your abdominal muscles tight. When your upper back reaches your seat back, reverse this motion and slowly return to an upright position. Repeat five times.

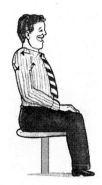

5. Shoulder Rolls

Duration: Five seconds. Begin by sitting tall. Keeping your arms relaxed, lift your shoulders up and back then roll them down and back. Repeat five times.

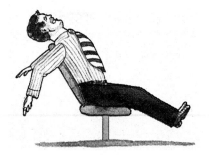

6. Chest and Neck Stretch

Duration: Five seconds. Begin by reclining against your seat back. Reach both arms out and allow them to slowly stretch open as you gently extend your head back. Straighten your legs out a bit at the same time. Hold for five seconds then slowly return to an upright position.

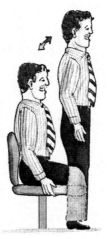

7. Sit-Stand Squats

Duration: Five seconds. Begin by sitting tall and facing front with both feet flat on the floor. Keeping your torso upright, stand up straight then sit down again. Repeat five times.

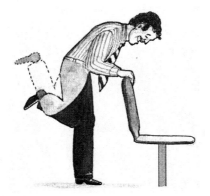

8. Bun Busters

Duration: Ten seconds. Begin by standing while holding the back of your chair. Step back and lean your upper body slightly forward toward the chair. Bend your right knee then extend your hip and slightly kick your leg back five times. Return your right foot to the floor and repeat on the left leg.

Range of Motion Stretching

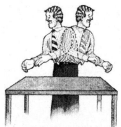

Turn your ribcage and head to one side at a time.

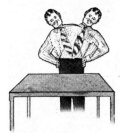

Tilt your ribcage and head to one side at a time.

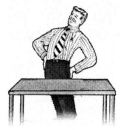

Arch your ribcage and head straight backward.

Figure 27. For a quick dose of mobility right at your desk, simply stand up where you are and take your spine through a gentle range of motion stretch by *slowly* turning right and then left, leaning to each side, and arching backwards. Only take each position as far as you can comfortably go. Hold momentarily at the endpoint of each stretch before moving on. This takes less than a minute.

Take a Deep Breath...

Another useful tip regarding motion and your body has to do with breathing. Seated deskwork is often associated with shallow respiration that uses the smaller breathing muscles of the upper back/neck region instead of the larger diaphragm muscle, located under the lungs in your lower ribcage. Shallow breathing leads to added muscle tightness in your neck and shoulders as you progressively hold greater tension in that area, which restricts the normal rising/falling motion of your ribcage.

To relieve tightness in the upper back/neck region, and to release tension in general, practice controlled breathing. When you fill your lungs with air and then empty them during respiration, your ribcage expands and contracts. Deep breathing is a way to mobilize your ribcage, particularly the tightest area in your upper back, located just below the base of your neck.

Practice the controlled breathing technique as follows:

1. Sit upright with correct posture
2. Slowly inhale deeply through your nose
3. Hold your breath for several seconds
4. Exhale completely through your mouth

Repeat this breathing cycle three times, each time breathing in a little deeper, holding your breath a little longer, and breathing out more completely. Practice this technique at least twice per day to help you relax.

"Sit Disc" Mobilization

The "sit disc" is a flat plastic circular disc about an inch in height and partially inflated with air. As you sit on the disc, your body weight can easily shift from front to back and side to side, 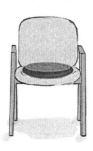 much the same as if you were sitting on a gym ball—but without the inconvenience of such a large object. You can perform the mobilization described below without a disc, but it is more difficult to do so. A "sit disc" supplier can be found using any Internet search engine.

To mobilize your spine, you will want to perform a circular motion in which your pelvis and ribcage are moving in opposite directions. The easiest way to start the mobilization is to simply move in separate side-to-side then front-to-back motions first before trying to combine the motions to complete a continuous circle.

Begin by shifting your pelvis to the left side while you simultaneously tilt your ribcage to the right (a). Then reverse the motion and shift your pelvis to the right side while you simultaneously tilt your ribcage to the left (b). Now move from side to side as you get familiar with that motion.

Next roll your pelvis back while you tilt your ribcage forward at the same time (c). Then reverse the motion and roll your pelvis forward while you tilt your ribcage back at the same time (d). Now move from front to back as you get familiar with that motion.

Finally, combine the motions so that your pelvis moves in a slow continuous circular fashion (left, back, right, front—left, back, right, front—) while your ribcage moves in the opposite circular motion as you have already practiced. You can then change the direction of rotation for diversity of movement. Perform this mobilization for one minute a couple of times a day at your desk.

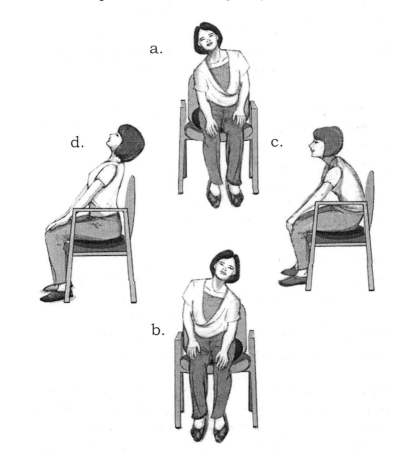

Get a Leg Up—Hamstring Stretch

As previously mentioned, people that sit a lot often have problems with the flexibility of their hamstring muscles. Tight hamstrings can cause poor sitting posture, and likewise, poor sitting posture can cause the hamstrings to get tight. The end result is that limitations will become evident with activities using the hamstring muscles such as forward bending, standing, walking, running, and climbing.

The connection between sitting posture and the hamstrings has to do with their attachment on the pelvis. The hamstring muscles attach to the "sit bones" or ischial tuberosities of the pelvis, as shown in Figure 28. If the hamstrings are tight, they pull on their attachment and encourage backward tilting of the pelvis, which flattens out the natural forward arch of the lower back. In the same way, prolonged sitting with poor posture, which rolls the pelvis backward, will decrease stretch on the hamstrings. Over time, the hamstring muscles will adapt by shortening to establish a new functional length. Then, when an activity is attempted that requires greater length from the hamstrings than sitting does, those tight muscles can restrict normal pelvic, hip, and knee motion and may cause significant problems.

The bottom line is that the hamstrings should be stretched regularly to help provide a better, more comfortable sitting position, as well as greater flexibility for everyday activities (Figure 29).

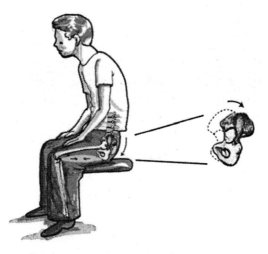

Figure 28. Tight hamstring muscles pull on their attachment at the bottom of the pelvis, tilting the pelvis backward, which rounds out the lower back.

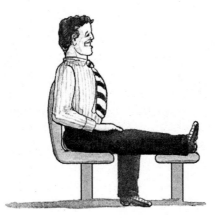

Figure 29. To stretch the hamstring muscles, sit up in a chair, fully into the seatback, and place one foot up on a surface in front of you that is about the same height as the seat bottom of your chair. Hold the stretch for 30 seconds for each leg at least twice per day.

Sitting: A Risk Factor

Fill up the gas tank in your car and you can drive until you run out of fuel. Charge your phone and talk until you are out of power. Machines are built for our convenience so that they work without the need for frequent maintenance. Some people would like to think that their bodies are machines and work in the same way. However, this is not the case. Living organisms, like ourselves, do require frequent mainte-nance. For example, you cannot eat one big meal and maintain your energy level without eating the rest of the day. You cannot take several extra deep breaths now to satisfy your need for breathing later. Nor can you sleep all weekend, then go without sleep during the week and expect to function normally. Our bodies have needs that must be met on an incremental basis, and these needs cannot be satisfied by doing more at one time to compensate for doing less or nothing at another time. A case in point is research which has shown that the negative effects of inactivity throughout the day cannot be reversed by one 30—60 minute exercise session when the rest of the day is highly sedentary. For healthy living, sitting time should be limited in the same way that people should limit their exposure to the sun or to secondhand smoke.

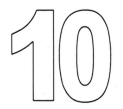

Practicing Good Posture

You should learn:

a. Why small imperfections in posture are significant over time
b. What the basic difference is between good and bad posture
c. How to properly align your body for most common activities

STEP TEN
Practicing Good Posture

Practicing good posture in everyday life involves one simple concept: Your spine has a normal shape, so position yourself during rest and activities to maintain that normal shape. The often-heard advice to "lift with your legs, not with your back" or "sit up straight" recommend that you keep the normal shape of your spine while lifting or sitting, because your back is stronger when it's not bent out of shape.

People get injured when lifting or during prolonged sitting because they bend or twist their spine out of position. Once you understand the proper neutral position for your spine and body, apply that understanding to your resting postures and activity positions. Your new posture awareness will play a vital role in reducing cumulative strain and preventing future problems.

Particularly with regard to sitting, people often fail to appreciate how minor postural faults can cause major trouble over time. To use an analogy, minor foot problems caused by an unsupportive insole or tight calf muscles probably wouldn't be noticed by someone who only needs to walk from the parking lot to the office and back each day, but would be a major issue for a marathon runner. As most of us are marathon sitters, what we sit on as well as how we sit really does matter. The small stresses and strains of poor posture that we take on daily can add up to large destructive forces before we know it—making good posture practice a priority.

Also remember that you need motion in your life. Periodically move the muscles and joints of your body throughout their available range of motion. Good posture practice, regular movement, and stretching can help you enjoy a lifetime of pain-free service from your spine.

The posture tips in this section illustrate proper positions for sitting and other common activities. For each activity, a correct and an incorrect example are shown. The correct postures show the body properly aligned to keep the normal shape; the incorrect postures show the body positioned so that the spine is bent out of its normal shape. This is always the difference between good and bad posture, no matter what the activity.

The POSTURE TIPS that follow include

• Basic sitting review
• Avoiding sitting on objects in your pocket
• Driving position
• Reclining position
• Reading position
• TV watching position
• Reading in bed
• Muscle effort with head-forward posture
• Parental warning about kids and video games
• Ergonomic workstation tune-up/checklist
• Standing postures
• Sleeping postures
• Talking on the phone
• Lifting technique

SITTING...

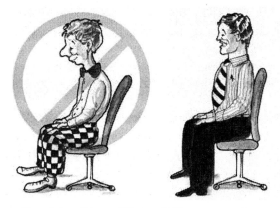

As described in Step Six, sitting requires that you bring your seatback to an upright position and lock it in place, scoot back fully into the seatback, and, ideally, place a lumbar support into the natural forward arch of your lower back.

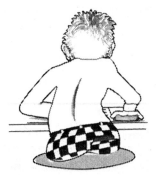

Avoid the habit of placing objects in the back pocket of your pants, such as a wallet, hairbrush, set of keys, cell phone, or makeup kit, which will raise one end of your pelvis and bend your back sideways, creating uneven pressures on your spine.

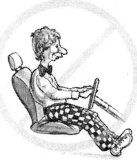 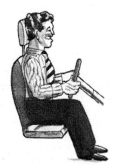

The proper driving position is similar to sitting in any other chair. Place your seatback upright to support your back and to keep your head close to the headrest. Fill the small space in the forward contour of your lower back with a small cushion or towel. Place your seat at a distance that allows your knees to bend at about hip level, with the steering wheel resting in your hands as your elbows are relaxed by your sides.

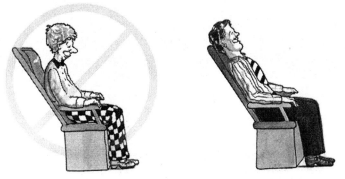

Keep your head in line with your back when you recline. Notice that the alignment between your head and shoulders should remain unchanged as you lower your seatback. Reclining is useful if you need to view something above head height, or just to rest, but it is otherwise a difficult position from which to work, read, eat or drink.

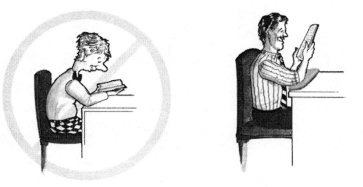

Bring all reading material—from the pages of a book to the display of a PDA, cell phone, or electronic game—up to your eye level because reading from the level of your lap or desktop requires forward bending of your head and neck. When your head drops down, the normal forward contour of your upper spine is bent out of shape, causing greater strain on your upper back and neck muscles that are holding up your head.

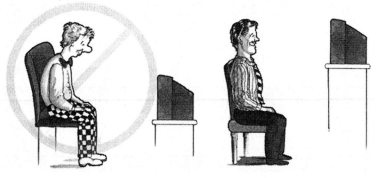

Move your TV or monitor to eye level. To position your head properly on your shoulders, keep your line of sight straight ahead. Place your TV or computer so that the top of the screen is at your eye level. If the glare of an overhead light is reflected onto the screen, slightly tilt the monitor.

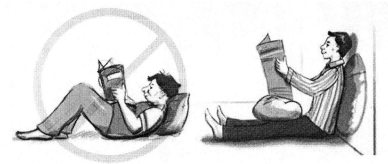

If you must read or watch TV in bed, instead of placing a large, bulky pillow under your head and thrusting your neck forward, support your back at a slight reclining angle against the wall. Make sure your head stays inline with your upper body. Reading material should be maintained at eye level, which may be aided by the use of another pillow on your lap to support the page bottoms.

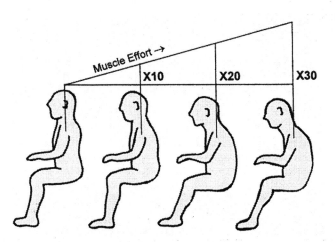

As shown above, muscle effort in the neck and upper back increases greatly for every inch your head travels forward, a good reason to always keep your head on straight!

KIDS AND VIDEO GAMES—A PARENTAL WARNING

As a result of the huge popularity of video games, on both large and small gaming consoles, more young people are preoccupied with this form of entertainment than ever before. In most instances, the kids clutching their portable gaming devices or handheld controllers are sitting in the worst of positions for prolonged periods of time, totally oblivious to the damage they are doing to themselves. Never before has there been a generation of youngsters who have subjected their developing bodies to this degree of long-term sedentary postural strain. We already know that general inactivity among today's youth over the past decade or so has led to an epidemic of obesity, but the spinal/orthopedic problems that will inevitably result from untold hours of rounded backs and protruding neck postures have yet to fully materialize.

It is only a matter of time, though, before problems will become evident, because a spine bent out of shape predictably wears at an accelerated rate. When this process begins at an early age, it leaves lots of time ahead for the further progression of degenerative disease. This matter is no less serious or less certain than the premature aging caused by repeated over-exposure of the skin to the sun. Parents should take the time to learn about proper body posture, help their kids understand the importance of avoiding undue postural strain, and give gentle reminders from time to time when they see their children have forgotten good posture practice.

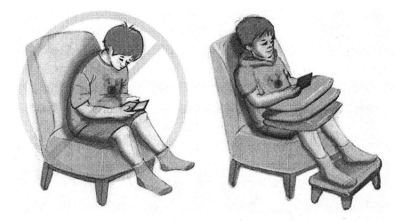

As with all sitting, the head and neck should be in line with the upper and lower back. Game consoles with video screens should be held slightly below eye level to avoid excessive forward head posture and neck bending that will occur when holding the console at lap level. The gaming device can be supported above the lap on a stack of pillows, on top of a backpack, or even on a cardboard box, to get the video screen closer to eye level and to allow the forearms a place to rest.

The natural separation between a person's line of sight (at or slightly below eye level) and the correct working position for their hands (about elbow height) cannot strictly be maintained, so a compromise has to be made by placing the game console at about the halfway point. In the case of larger consoles where the images are displayed directly onto regular TV screens, upright sitting with the back well supported and the controller held on the lap or just above lap level on a small pillow is the correct posture.

STEP BY STEP ERGONOMIC TUNE-UP...

1. Your first step in tuning up your workstation is to sit up correctly in your chair. Next, completely relax your arm by your side (a). Without tensing your muscles or elevating your shoulder, bend your elbow so that your forearm is parallel with the floor (b). This establishes the proper working position for your hands, which aligns your hands with your forearms and avoids excessive up and down or side to side bending of your wrists.

2. With your elbows relaxed by your sides and your hands at their proper working position at about elbow height, the correct keyboard and mouse location should accommodate this hand position. That means your desktop should be at elbow level. If your desktop is too high, then use a pull-out tray to lower your keyboard and mouse, or raise your chair and rest your feet on a footrest. Consider bringing your mouse hand closer to your body by using a shorter keyboard (with a separate 10-key pad), and move your mouse pad closer to the center of your body, as described below in Step By Step #6.

3. Arrange your desktop so that your monitor is centered on your sitting position. If you frequently work with paper documents, use a document holder to place your papers next to the monitor at eye level, or at least on a clipboard between your monitor and keyboard, for easier viewing. The worst place to read from is the desktop level. Put frequently used items, such as the phone, a cup, or a calculator, within easy reach of your arms.

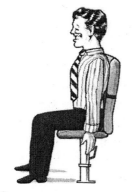

a.

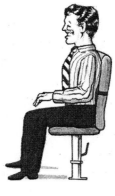

b.

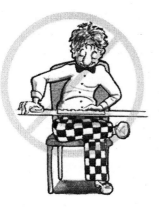

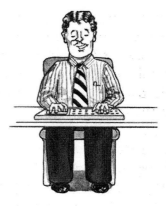

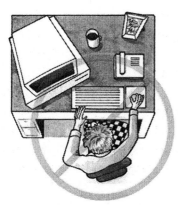

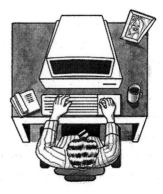

4. Place your monitor so that the top of the screen is at your eye level and within a distance that you can touch with your fingertips when your arm is extended straight ahead. You may use an armrest to help support your forearms; however, only a portion of your arm weight should be supported by the armrest to reduce pressure at the underside of your elbow and to allow full motion of your arm and shoulder. The forward edge of your seat should be about three fingers' width away from the back of your knees as you sit.

5. Notice that the natural separation between your line of sight and the correct working position for your hands can be maintained with the proper desktop setup (b), but not with the standard laptop setup (a). If you often use a laptop, it is *highly recommended* that you get a laptop holder to elevate your screen and use an external mouse and keyboard. Other useful items that may help you to sit and work more comfortably include fully adjustable chairs, lumbar supports, footrests, pullout trays, document holders, telephone headsets, monitor risers, and sit-stand workstations.

6. Most people position the keyboard, including the alphanumeric keys and the numeric ten-key portion, to their center, and then off-center the mouse to one side (a). If you do not use the ten-key portion as often as the regular typing keys, consider installing a "short" keyboard with a separate ten-key pad. Then move the mouse (or other pointing device) to the edge of the keyboard, center the keyboard and mouse together, and place the 10-key pad alongside the mouse (b).

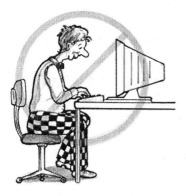

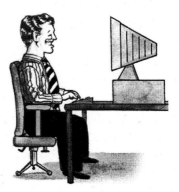

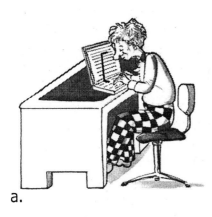

a.

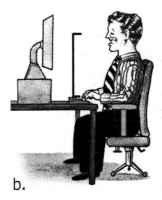

b.

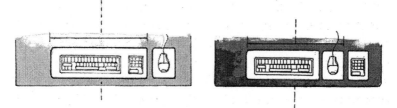

a.

b.

7. More effort is required to move the mouse using only wrist motion than to move it a similar distance using full upper arm motion. Normal upper extremity movement during keyboard and mouse use should involve all the joints of the arm and hand to minimize strain on any one part, so remember to sit upright in a relaxed and supported posture to allow freedom of movement from your shoulders down to your fingers.

8. Bringing your mouse or other pointing device in toward your center and down toward your lap is important because it affects shoulder elevation. Working at the computer for long periods of time can cause muscle, joint, and nerve problems if you elevate your shoulder and reach out with your arm. Holding your arm out and away from your body during sitting deskwork *is no different* than standing or walking around with your arm held up and out. Demonstrate that to yourself now by first relaxing your arm by your side, then raising your arm several inches up and away from your body. That "up-and-away" arm position quickly becomes uncomfortable because your neck and shoulder muscles have to support the entire weight of your arm. It is much better to work with your upper arms hanging loosely by your sides while your elbows are bent such that your forearms are roughly parallel with the floor. This position requires that your keyboard and mouse (or other device) be located close enough to your body to allow your elbows to rest directly under your shoulders when sitting. Modify the arrangement of your keyboard and mouse to accomplish this as described earlier.

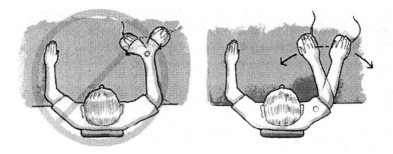

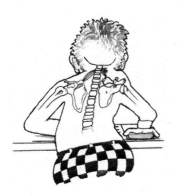 =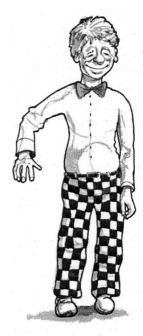

Workstation Ergonomic Tune-Up Checklist

Your Chair

❑   The seatback of the chair is set to an upright, nearly vertical position and locked into place. A lumbar support that fills the natural forward arch of your lower back is placed just above the beltline of your waist.

❑   The chair height allows your feet to rest comfortably flat on the floor with your knees at or slightly below hip level.

❑   The bottom of the chair is the correct size to allow you to sit back fully against the seatback yet also maintain a three-finger distance between the front edge of the seat and the back of your knees.

❑   If your seat bottom tilts, slope the front of the seat downward a few degrees if desired.

❑   The armrests, if any, are set low to support a portion of your arm weight but do not limit free motion of your arms during keyboarding, mouse/pointing device use, or writing.

Your Desk

❑   The desktop is ideally set at your elbow level. A pull-out tray can be used to place your keyboard and mouse/pointing device at your proper working height as described in Step By Step Ergonomic Tune-Up #1, which also relaxes your arms by your sides and places your hands directly in front of you.

❑ You avoid using a death grip on your mouse or other pointing device, or depressing the keys with unnecessary force while typing. Replace the keyboard or mouse if they do not respond to light touch inputs.

❑ The items you use most frequently, such as a telephone, notepad, drinking cup, pen/pencil, or file folders, are within an easy arm's reach.

Your Monitor

❑ Your monitor is located directly in front of you, approximately at arm's length. You can change the resolution of the monitor to enlarge or reduce image and font size as needed.

❑ The top of the monitor's screen is at your eye level (below eye level if you wear bifocals). At an arm's length distance from the screen, your field of vision covers the entire screen without having to bend your head down.

❑ The screen is tilted back a few degrees at the top for easier viewing as desired. If the screen is reflecting any glare, the monitor position is shifted slightly or an antiglare filter is fitted over the screen.

❑ You are working under adequate lighting for the tasks you perform. You focus on distant objects every so often when working on the computer for extended periods of time to reduce eyestrain.

BEYOND SITTING

STANDING...

When standing and bending or leaning forward to perform any task, give yourself a helping hand by extending an arm down to provide added support. This decreases the strain on your lower back by reducing the effort of the spinal muscles needed to counteract the extra weight of your body leaning forward.

Stand and walk as if a string were pulling you up from your breast bone (the top front of your ribcage). Avoid the hallmark of poor posture, which is a sunken chest. For the most part, you will correct the posture of your head, shoulders, and lower back by maintaining an upright ribcage. Be aware that your feet can also affect your posture. Like the spine, the foot also has structural arches that need support. Because the hard surfaces we most often stand and walk on tend to flatten the foot, consider using an upgraded insole in your shoes to provide the proper arch support. These insoles are available at most sporting goods stores.

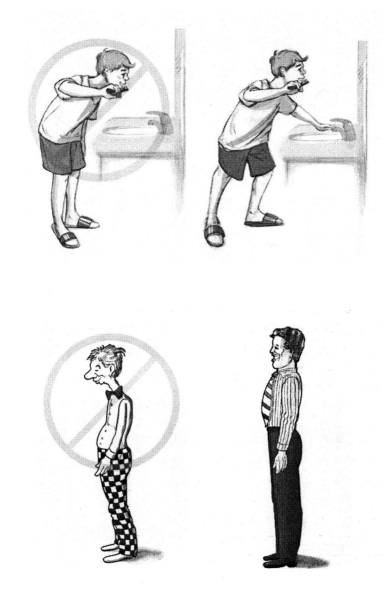

SLEEPING...

When lying down on your back, support your *neck* with a small pillow rather than sticking a large, bulky pillow under your head. This keeps your head in alignment with the rest of your body and helps to maintain the natural forward contour of your neck.

When lying down on your side, support your *head* with a pillow that fills the space between your mattress and your ear so that your head stays in the midline of your body. Avoid tucking your chin. Instead, maintain a relaxed distance between your chin and chest.

Sleep on your back with a pillow under your knees or on your side with a pillow between your knees to support and relax your lower back.

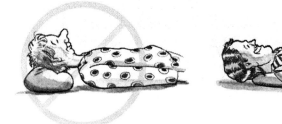

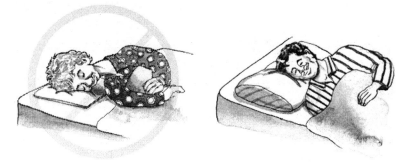

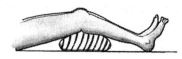

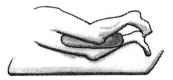

OTHER TASKS...

Wear a headset for frequent or long phone calls, at the office, at home, or when mobile. Holding the phone between your ear and shoulder strains the muscles in your neck/shoulder area and bends your spine out of shape. If you repeatedly cradle the phone toward one side, your neck will be thrown out of balance, eventually causing injury and pain. Using a headset also frees your arms and hands for deskwork, chores, driving, or just relaxing.

As you lift objects, keep them as close to your body as possible and at the midline of your body, optimally about at the level of your belly button. Keep your back from rounding forward by using leg strength to lift. Avoid twisting or bending at the waist by using your whole body to turn if you must move to the right or left side. The danger zones in lifting are below knee level and above shoulder level, so be extra careful or get help when lifting down low or up high. Try stacking objects that need lifting on top of a box or cart instead of on the ground. Use a stepladder to reach or shelve high objects. Remember that even small or light objects can cause serious back injury if your lifting posture is incorrect.

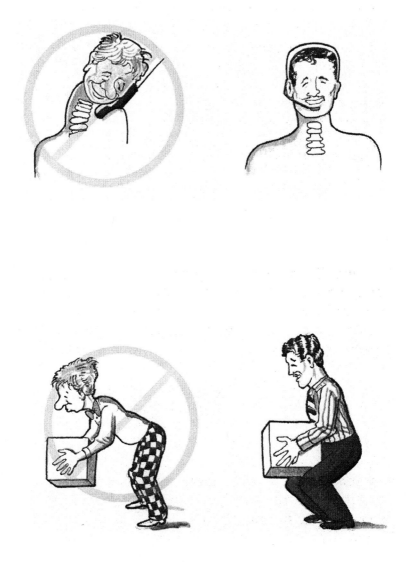

Posture   1. The way in which one is placed or arranged. 2. A frame of mind affecting one's thoughts or behavior. 3. The way in which a person holds or carries his or her body.

Roget's II: The New Thesaurus, Third Edition

posture
noun[1]: stance, carriage, pose
noun[2]: beliefs, feeling, mood
verb: attitudinize, display, masquerade

Roget's II: New Millennium Thesaurus, First Edition

In Review

A concise summary of the ten steps to looking
and feeling better with good posture

IN REVIEW...

STEP ONE
A healthy spine is specifically shaped to maximize strength and flexibility. When the body is in a neutral position, that normal shape is outwardly expressed as good posture.

STEP TWO
The spinal bones, or vertebrae, are held in place by connective soft tissue structures that play a major role in determining the shape and mobility of the spine.

STEP THREE
Poor posture habits, over time, strain the connective soft tissues and bend the spine out of its normal shape, making it increasingly difficult to stand or sit up straight.

STEP FOUR
When the spine is bent out of its normal shape, the vertebrae and connective soft tissues wear unevenly and become increasingly hardened by the process of degeneration.

STEP FIVE
When you are standing or sitting in a neutral position, a natural forward arch, the lumbar lordosis, is normally present in the lower back area of your spine.

STEP SIX
Good sitting posture involves keeping your body erect by scooting your buttocks back against your seatback, locking your seatback in an upright position, and supporting the natural forward arch in your lower back.

STEP SEVEN

Slumping is a bad habit that creates fatigue, increases the risk of repetitive strain and sports injury, and may result in permanent deformity. Use visual reminders, ergonomic devices, and other tools to maintain your good posture practice and avoid slumping.

STEP EIGHT

Improper sitting or long periods of deskwork cause the body to become rounded forward. Extension stretching can help you relax tight postural muscles and regain a healthier spinal position.

STEP NINE

When you sit for long periods of time, your body's systems become idle. Periodic motion and stretching of moderate intensity can help recharge your breathing and blood flow to keep you alert and flexible.

STEP TEN

Good posture practice is an ongoing awareness of the normal shape of your spine, maintaining a neutral position during rest and activity, and satisfying your body's recurring need for motion.

The Bottom Line

Poor sitting posture is bad for your health, correct sitting posture is good for your health, and not sitting for long is best for your health.

Unless some misfortune has made it impossible, everyone can have good posture.

Loretta Young

I want to get old gracefully. I want to have good posture, I want to be healthy and be an example to my children.

Sting

Some Final Thoughts

A wrap-up of the benefits good posture
practice brings and research that supports it

SOME FINAL THOUGHTS

In today's culture, little emphasis is placed on posture (or poise, as it has been called in past generations). In fact, slumping has become so commonplace that the detrimental effects of poor posture are often overlooked as some of the most frequent causes of current and future problems. That's a definite step backward for our health. The basis for healthy living and graceful aging will always include such simple concepts as a wholesome diet, regular exercise, adequate rest, attention to posture to care for the body's frame, and a positive outlook on life.

Regarding symptoms of health problems, remember that you usually have to accumulate a certain level of damage before you start feeling any pain. Therefore, having no discomfort at the moment does not ensure that an underlying problem isn't developing, nor does relief from pain necessarily mean that an injury is completely resolved. The best lifelong approach is to remain proactive and practice good posture as a habit, regardless of symptoms, to preserve the structure and function of your body's frame. Whatever your condition, improving your posture will contribute to improving your health.

The benefits of practicing good posture far outweigh the extra effort it takes to properly maintain the normal shape of your spine during activities and resting positions. Those benefits include

✓Looking younger ✓Reducing fatigue ✓Breathing easier ✓Maintaining height ✓Moving more freely ✓Avoiding pain ✓Preventing injury ✓ Minimizing degeneration

Consistent posture awareness not only makes good common sense, it is also supported by research. Studies confirm that the proper sitting position is more comfortable and healthier than slumping. Although most people tend to have their favorite chairs and sitting styles, we know from the study of human anatomy and ergonomics that certain postures are healthier than others for supporting the weight of the body when seated. Those proper postures are described in detail in Step Six (correct sitting), Step Ten (posture tips), and The Seated Spine (Appendix E). Less clear are the contributing factors that tend to make people feel comfortable while sitting. Interestingly, researchers have concluded that comfort in a seated position is the absence of discomfort; that is, a comfortable person is simply unaware of pain or tiredness from sitting.

The following is a summary of contributing factors that have been tested and found related to greater sitting comfort:
• A seat that provides a backrest with a better fit to the shape of the body
• A seat that provides a backrest with contact to both the upper and lower back
• A seat that provides the most even pressure distribution for the back and buttock areas
• A seated posture with less forward leaning at the waist

• A seated posture with less neck, shoulder, and back muscle activity
• A seated posture with less slumping (less stature loss)

As it turns out, these factors related to sitting comfort are all perfectly matched to the proper sitting posture presented in this book. Sitting well back into your chair with your seatback upright and the natural forward curve of your lower back supported, your feet flat on the floor or footrest, and your monitor or reading material at eye level is the most correct and comfortable seated position.

The natural forward curve of the lower back, called the "lumbar lordosis," has also been linked to a person's overall well-being. Research into the effects of abnormal spinal curves on a person's physical status and mental outlook found that loss of lumbar lordosis was directly related to lower social functioning and reduced general health. Considering the stiffness and tightness that results from degenerative changes in a spine that is bent out of shape, as described in Step Four, and the weakness and instability created in a spine that is lacking the normal contours, as described in Step Five, these research findings are not surprising.

The Science of Sitting confirms that you can look and feel better with good posture. Combine that with the movement and stretching tips found in Step Nine, and you'll be that rare swan in an otherwise crowded world of ducklings.

APPENDIX

The content of the book up to this point has consisted of need-to-know information crucial for your understanding and practice of good posture. The sections that follow build on that foundation of knowledge with greater depth, details, and insights into the subject of sitting posture, and contain valuable tools to support and further advance your posture IQ and healthier lifestyle.

A. Checking and Recording Your Own Posture

B. Monitor Placard and Instructions: A visual reference to help with good posture practices

C. Weekly Self-Care Record Form and Instructions

D. About Gravity

E. The Seated Spine

F. Injury Prevention

G. Winning the Battle with Back Pain

A. Checking and recording your own posture

You can get a basic idea about the shape of your own spine by looking closely at your posture in a mirror. To check your posture from the front view, it is best to use a full-length mirror mounted on a wall or door. Taping one string that runs straight down the center of the mirror, and two that run straight across from side to side (one about shoulder height, one about hip height), will make viewing your posture a bit easier. To position yourself correctly when checking posture, stand centered in front of the mirror, at a distance that allows you to see as much of your body as possible. Your feet should be about shoulder-width apart with your weight evenly distributed (Figure 30).

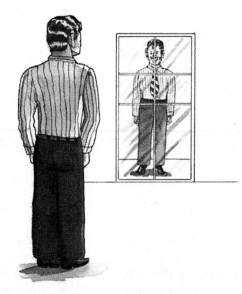

Figure 30. Checking your posture in the mirror

Close your eyes for a few moments to let yourself settle comfortably into a natural stance, as if you were standing in line. Then open your eyes, being careful not to move any part of your body (except for your eyes, of course). Look closely at your posture from the top down. Ideally, the line in the mirror (or an imaginary line) should run straight down the middle of your body. Your shoulders and hips should be level (as in Figure 31). If not, see if you notice any of the common posture problems listed on the next page. Record your results by marking each box that applies.

Checking your posture from a side view requires the help of another person (since you can't see your own side posture without turning your head to look in the mirror). Position yourself as you did when checking your posture from the front. Ask your helper to stand off to your side, at about the same distance from you as you are standing from the mirror.

Ideally, your head, mid-body, and lower body should be vertically aligned so that an imaginary line would run through the middle of your ear, your shoulder top, your hip, and your ankle (as in Figure 32). If not, see if your helper notices any of the common posture problems listed. Record your results by marking each box that applies.

Another helpful idea is to have a picture taken of your natural stance from the front and side views. You could then draw-in the vertical lines running down from the top of your body to create an accurate record of any postural imbalances.

Common Posture Problems Checklist (front view)

Your head

- ❑ If your head is turned, you'll see more of one side of your face than the other side.
- ❑ If your head is tilted, you'll see your chin slightly pointing to one side instead of straight down.
- ❑ If your head is off-center, you'll see your neck slanted more toward one side of your body.

Your midbody (ribcage area)

- ❑ If your midbody is turned, you'll see one shoulder and/or one hand hanging farther forward than the one on the other side.
- ❑ If your midbody is tilted, you'll see one shoulder and/or one hand hanging higher than the one on the other side.
- ❑ If your midbody is off-center, you'll see a greater space between your arm and waist on one side than on the other side.

Your lower body (pelvis area and legs)

- ❑ If your lower body is turned, you'll see one hip farther forward than the one on the other side.
- ❑ If your lower-body is off-center, you'll see that your legs are not parallel.

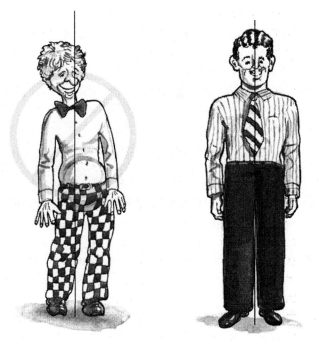

Figure 31. Front view of poor vs. good posture

Common Posture Problems Checklist (side view)

Your head

❑ If your head is forward, the middle of your ear will be in front of your shoulder top.

Your midbody (ribcage area)

❑ If your midbody is leaning backward, your shoulder top will be behind your hip.

❑ If your midbody is leaning forward, your shoulder top will be in front of your hip.

❑ If your ribcage is rounded, your spine will have a greater backward curvature or "hunchback" in the mid-back area.

Your lower body (pelvis area and legs)

❑ If your lower body is forward, your hip will be in front of your ankles.

❑ If your pelvis is tilted down, your spine will have a greater forward curvature or "swayback" in the lower back area.

After checking your posture, if you've noticed any of the common posture problems, your results suggest that your spine has changed from its normal shape. Follow the steps in this book to help you understand how and why a healthier spine and posture is both possible and essential.

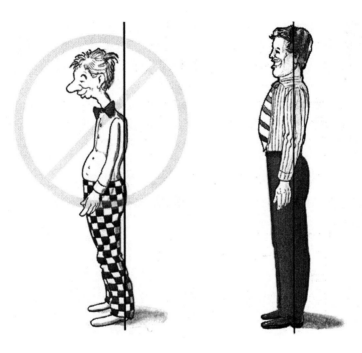

Figure 32. Side view of poor vs. good posture

B. Monitor Placard and Instructions: A visual reference to help with good posture practices

The placard is for you to place on your computer monitor or any other convenient place where it's helpful to have a visual reminder of good posture. Remove the placard from the back cover of this book, place an adhesive (such as double-sided tape) on the back of the placard, and then stick the placard on a clean, flat surface. Alternatively, the placard may simply be used as a bookmark.

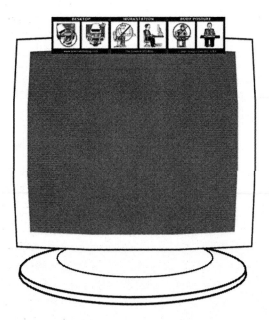

C. Weekly Self-Care Record

The Weekly Self-Care Record (p. 130) is an easy way to track the simple stretch and movement tips presented in this book. Although you may sincerely intend to make use of preventive measures to stay healthy and alert, it is all too easy to forget when you get busy or tired. Keeping a record reminds you what to do and what you have actually done.

These instructions describe the purpose of each column in the Weekly Self-Care Record:

1. Write the month and date in numbered format (for example, 10/01 for October first) in the box with the correct day of the week.

2. Perform the neck/back extension stretch 10—15 minutes each day, as described in Step Eight. Check the box after completing the stretch.

3. Perform some form of general activity such as brisk walking or stair climbing three times per day in five-minute increments. The activities described in this item, along with those described in items 4 and 5 below, should provide you with a good diversity of motion. Check the appropriate box after completing each activity session.

4. The Sixty Second Workout (p. 76—79) is a series of eight exercises/stretches that can be performed, in whole or in part, at your desk as a quick way to add motion to your life. Check the appropriate

box after completing all or part of the workout. If you perform part of the workout, write the number (1-8) of the exercise(s) or stretch(es) you did in the comments section.

5. The standing Range Of Motion (ROM) stretch, done right at your desk (p. 80), is another quick and very convenient method for adding body movement into your day. Periodically, you can alternate the standing ROM with mobilization of your spine while in a sitting position (p. 82–83). This is easy to accomplish on a Sit Disc and takes no extra time away from your work. Switch between the standing ROM and the Sit Disc mobilization for variety, and check the box after completing one set of ROM or mobilization stretches.

6. Leg stretching (p. 84) only requires that you pull up an adjacent chair of similar height to rest your foot on. This simple but highly effective activity should be repeated twice per day. Check off the box following your AM and PM stretches.

7. Perform deep breathing (p. 81) at least twice per day to mobilize the ribcage, get more oxygen into the body, and relieve stress. Check the appropriate box after performing each set of three consecutive cycles of deep breathing.

8. Check the box indicating the level of your workload as you perceive it.

9. Check the box indicating your overall stress level as you define it.

10. If you are aware of any discomfort such as pain, fatigue, tightness, or stiffness, indicate the status of those symptoms.

11. The comments section is for giving feedback, noting trends, or recording ideas. For example, you might write "shoulder rolls (#6) in Sixty Second Workout felt particularly good" or "take time for deep breathing and standing ROM more often—it helps."

Correlation

If you are consistent in making daily entries into the Self-Care Record Form, you will likely discover certain patterns involving symptoms and situations. For most people there is a definite connection between increased work, increased stress, and increased pain. This is partly due to simple time constraints, given that there is usually less time to rest, stretch, and alternate tasks with heavy workloads and overtime hours, when in fact these circumstances necessitate more attention to self-care, not less. The other part of the correlation has to do with mental or emotional fatigue that significantly lowers our threshold for dealing with any kind of physical discomfort. These factors acting together are often the cause of repeated episodes of pain. Breaking the cycle requires that you practice brief but regular self-care techniques to offset cumulative strain before it recurrently reaches critical levels.

A Weekly Self-Care Record Form is located on the next page. Make copies (or download the form) as needed to keep track of your progress.

Weekly Self-Care Record

Date Month/Day	Neck/back Extension Stretch	Stairs or Brisk Walking	Sixty Second Workout	Standing ROM or Sit Disc	Hamstring Stretching	Deep Breathing	Workload	Stress Level	Symptom Status	Comments
Monday	10-15 min. □	□ AM □ Noon □ PM	□ AM □ Noon □ PM	□ AM □ Noon □ PM	□ AM □ Noon □ PM	□ AM □ Noon □ PM	□ Light □ Moderate □ Heavy	□ Low □ Med □ High	□ Same □ Better □ Worse	
Tuesday	10-15 min. □	□ AM □ Noon □ PM	□ AM □ Noon □ PM	□ AM □ Noon □ PM	□ AM □ Noon □ PM	□ AM □ Noon □ PM	□ Light □ Moderate □ Heavy	□ Low □ Med □ High	□ Same □ Better □ Worse	
Wednesday	10-15 min. □	□ AM □ Noon □ PM	□ AM □ Noon □ PM	□ AM □ Noon □ PM	□ AM □ Noon □ PM	□ AM □ Noon □ PM	□ Light □ Moderate □ Heavy	□ Low □ Med □ High	□ Same □ Better □ Worse	
Thursday	10-15 min. □	□ AM □ Noon □ PM	□ AM □ Noon □ PM	□ AM □ Noon □ PM	□ AM □ Noon □ PM	□ AM □ Noon □ PM	□ Light □ Moderate □ Heavy	□ Low □ Med □ High	□ Same □ Better □ Worse	
Friday	10-15 min. □	□ AM □ Noon □ PM	□ AM □ Noon □ PM	□ AM □ Noon □ PM	□ AM □ Noon □ PM	□ AM □ Noon □ PM	□ Light □ Moderate □ Heavy	□ Low □ Med □ High	□ Same □ Better □ Worse	
Saturday	10-15 min. □	□ AM □ Noon □ PM	□ AM □ Noon □ PM	□ AM □ Noon □ PM	□ AM □ Noon □ PM	□ AM □ Noon □ PM	□ Light □ Moderate □ Heavy	□ Low □ Med □ High	□ Same □ Better □ Worse	
Sunday	10-15 min. □	□ AM □ Noon □ PM	□ AM □ Noon □ PM	□ AM □ Noon □ PM	□ AM □ Noon □ PM	□ AM □ Noon □ PM	□ Light □ Moderate □ Heavy	□ Low □ Med □ High	□ Same □ Better □ Worse	

The Weekly Self-Care Record is downloadable as a Word document or PDF file at The Science of Sitting website: www.scienceofsitting.com

D. About Gravity

We spend our entire lifetimes interacting with the
natural environment and its variations of air
temperature, pressure and humidity, heat, light,
radiation, and electromagnetism. One of the
invariables in our existence on Earth is gravity,
and just because it is constant we seldom think
about it, except perhaps indirectly if we happen to
trip and fall, drop something, or walk up a steep
hill. However, gravity plays a very significant role
in human anatomy and physiology during a
person's lifetime, and ultimately it is the reason
we need to be concerned about posture.

We know from observations of those relatively few
people who have escaped Earth's gravity what
happens to the human body in the weightlessness
of space. Astronauts experience problems with
motion sickness due to inner ear dysfunction,
fluid shifts out of the lower extremities and into
the head that cause "Bird Legs" and "Puffy Face
Syndrome," considerable muscle and bone wasting,
elongation of the spine, cardiovascular decondi-
tioning, and digestive irregularities.

This information tells us that gravity is important
for the maintenance of our normal spatial
orientation, body fluid balance, muscle mass,
bone density, spinal contours, heart and lung
conditioning, and digestive function. On the
other hand, in the absence of gravitational
(weight-bearing) forces, any position that doesn't
violate normal ranges of body motion is just as
good as any other, and posture therefore becomes

irrelevant. So it is gravity that actually makes posture important.

What exactly is gravity? Gravity is a force of attraction that exists between any two objects, which is determined by the size and distance of the objects. What that means in practical terms is that you are constantly being pulled (accelerated) toward the center of the Earth. The Earth is also being pulled toward you, but because Earth's mass (amount of matter) compared to your mass is immensely greater, your effect on the Earth is negligible.

Weight is a byproduct of gravity that gives a measure of the force with which you are being pulled toward the Earth. Larger people weigh more because the law of gravity says the greater the mass, the stronger the gravitational force of attraction. For this same reason, your weight as measured on the moon would be much less because the moon has a smaller mass than the Earth.

The force of gravity at sea level on Earth is commonly called 1"g". That 1"g" is responsible for your need of a complex bone, muscle, and connective tissue system to hold you upright and resist your downfall toward the Earth. As you sit you are being pulled downward into your chair, which is therefore pushing upward against your body, resulting in compression, tension, and shear forces acting on your spine.

These forces cause a ½"—¾" daily shrinkage of body height due to moisture loss in the discs of your spine. Most of this shrinkage is recovered overnight as you sleep (horizontally), but most people will permanently lose ½" to 2" in height from this recurring process over the course of a lifetime. You can manage gravity and the resultant forces acting on your body efficiently or inefficiently according to your posture habits, and then enjoy the benefits or suffer the consequences that will surely follow.

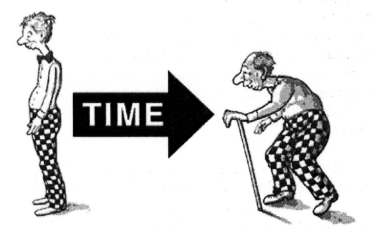

Poor posture always loses the fight against gravity.

E. The Seated Spine

Sitting is an important subject of scientific study because deviations from neutral posture over long periods have been shown to be associated with back and neck pain, disc degeneration, risk of arthritis, and muscle spasms, not to mention workplace injury and lost productivity with the related costs of treatment and disability. In fact, about 100 million workdays are lost each year in the U.S. due to lower back pain, more of which is related to sitting than ever before.

Sitting correctly is a balance of several interrelated factors including weight distribution, muscle activity, disc compression, joint pressure, spinal cord tension, neutral spine alignment, and (of course) comfort. A lot of research has gone into understanding what happens to the human body in the sitting position. Although different interprettations of the research do exist, there is enough of a consensus to reach some important conclusions and to make some solid recommendations.

The science of sitting ultimately comes down to gravity. The compressive force of gravity must be efficiently managed by the body structures to avoid certain injury. Those body structures primarily consist of ① spinal bones (or vertebrae) including the ② vertebral body, ③ interconnecting articular facet joints, and ④ intervertebral disc, as well as the muscles and connective tissues. With proper sitting posture, the body's weight is evenly distributed so that no one structure is overloaded.

On the other hand, improper sitting causes a focus of pressure and the premature breakdown of body structures under greater loads.

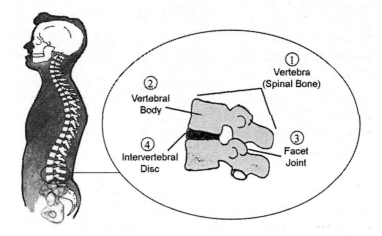

There are actually different correct sitting postures depending on whether you are working or just resting. Working posture implies that you need your head upright to give you a field of vision at desk level, as with computer work, writing, drawing, and most reading. Resting posture implies your head can be reclined in line with your back as with napping, listening to music, or watching a big screen movie.

Correct sitting in all cases relies on the support of the normal forward arch of the lower back (called the lumbar lordosis). The lumbar lordosis spans across all five lumbar vertebrae and exists mostly because of the shape of the intervertebral discs. The discs are thicker and taller toward their front portion and thinner and shorter toward their back portion, making the discs wedge shaped.

With the lower back contoured into the proper lumbar lordosis, the discs maintain their normal wedge shape, and weight of the upper body is correctly distributed through the lumbar spine onto a) the vertebral bodies, b) the intervertebral discs, and c) the facet joints. At each level of the lumbar spine the vertebral bodies, intervertebral discs, and facet joints act together with the connective soft tissues to resist the resultant forces of compression, tension, and shear we experience with everyday activities.

Measurements of pressure in the lower spine discs have shown that lumbar lordosis is inversely proportional to intradiscal pressure. That means there is less disc compression when there is more lower back arch. The wedge shape of the disc when the lumbar spine is in lordosis is what accounts for the decrease in disc pressure.

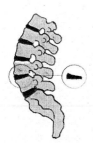 Lumbar disc pressure along with activity of the back muscles change with different sitting positions. The lowest disc pressures and muscle activity measured during experiments have been obtained when the lumbar spine was extended backward over a backrest.

Disc pressure is important because the ability of the disc to act as a hydrostatic (non-moving fluid) cushion depends on a high water content, which is lost in forward flexed postures that change the disc shape and round the lower back. Therefore, in the absence of lumbar lordosis, the lower back flattens or rounds outward, increasing disc pressure and decreasing the disc's ability to act as a hydrostatic cushion to absorb/disperse forces.

Loss of water content, or dehydration, in the lumbar discs decreases the disc height and increases loading of the interconnecting spinal facet joints. The narrowing that occurs with decreased disc height along with the resultant increase in pressure across the facet joints can cause damage and produce pain. Good evidence shows that the lumbar facet joints are capable of bearing vertical compressive loads along the spinal column. While the vertebral body and the inter-vertebral disc are considered to be the principal load-bearing components of the spine, the lumbar articular facets have been shown to carry 3—25% of the spine's compressive load.

One study found that in very slight extension the lumbar facet joints carried between 10 and 40% of the applied compressive force, while another study found that in erect standing the facets uphold about 16% of the compressive force. If the facet joint is arthritic, the load can become as high as 47%, indicating that an increase in facet load due to disc narrowing can be a cause of osteoarthritis (wear and tear) in the spine.

So far we have learned that lumbar lordosis is important for sitting because when the lower back is positioned with the correct forward contour the normal disc shape is preserved, disc pressure is minimized, disc hydration and disc height are maintained, and weight-bearing pressure through the facet joints is properly distributed.

Muscle activity in the lower back, as was previously mentioned, is also reduced in sitting or standing postures with the lumbar lordosis intact because the weight of the upper body projecting downward falls closer to the center of the lower spine. The distance from any point of rotation on the spine and a force acting on it is called a lever arm. Those forces would include a) the weight of the upper body itself, plus anything a person also happens to be holding or lifting, and b) the pull of the back muscles. While the lever arm B between the lower back muscles and the lumbar spine is more or less a fixed distance, the lever arm A between the upper body and the lumbar spine can increase significantly with forward bending, as shown below:

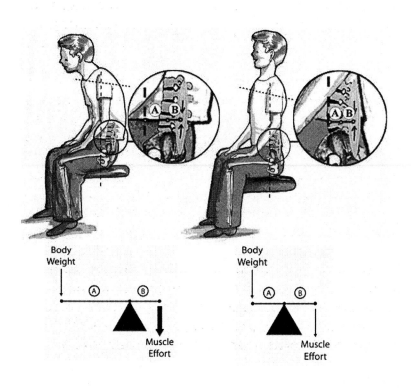

In upright gravity-dependant positions such as sitting and standing, when the upper body weight increases in distance away from the center of the lower spine, the forward bending force acting on the spine is sharply increased—so the back muscles must exert a greater effort to resist the added force. Therefore, rounding of the lower spine and forward bending of the upper spine (slumping) isn't really relaxing at all for the back muscles.

It is also known that the position of the head on the body is significantly affected by sitting postures and the lumbar lordosis. The bones of the neck (cervical vertebrae) are also normally contoured in a forward arch (cervical lordosis). If the lower back rounds out when sitting, the ribcage will drop down and forward, resulting in neck flexion and anterior head carriage. Thus the postural tendency is that seated loss of lumbar spine *and* cervical spine lordosis occur at the same time. Loss of cervical lordosis causes an increase in cervical disc pressure, an increase in muscle activity in the neck muscles, and tension on the spinal cord, brain stem, and nerve roots. It is therefore not surprising that a lumbar support to promote lumbar lordosis has been shown to reduce anterior head carriage as well as low back pain.

Unfortunately, most people demonstrate a significant loss of lumbar lordosis in seated compared to standing postures. Sitting often encourages backward tilting of the pelvis with a concurrent reduction of the lumbar lordosis,

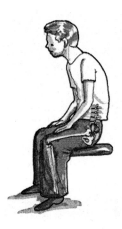

increase in muscle tension, disc compression, and pressure on the ischial tuberosities (the sit bones). Unsupported sitting with the lower spine rounded out places the body's weight directly over the ischial tuberosities, causing a highly focused pressure distribution (tissue compression) at the sit bones. The area directly under the ischial tuberosities makes up only 8% of the seat surface but carries up to 65% of the body weight. To distribute weight and pressure more effectively, a chair's seatback and lumbar support must be properly positioned so that a portion of the body weight is directed horizontally into the seatback to diffuse vertical compression at the ischial tuberosities. Sitting with the feet flat on the floor and the upper extremity weight partially supported by armrests also helps a bit to reduce a focus of compression at the ischial tuberosities.

There has been much written about the so-called thigh/trunk angle. In standard upright sitting, the angle between the thigh (which is horizontal) and the trunk (which is vertical) is about 90 degrees. It has been suggested that opening the thigh/trunk angle to 110—135 degrees during sitting can decrease disc pressures in the lumbar spine. The problem with an open thigh/trunk angle is that either the seatback must be significantly reclined, or the seat bottom must be sharply angled downward. Significantly reclining

the seatback for working
posture results in an
undesirable compensatory
forward flexion angle of the
head and neck to maintain
a field of vision at desk level,
as shown here.

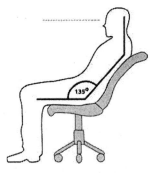

Sharply angling the seat bottom downward would
result in forward sliding off the chair. There is a
useful two-part seat bottom design that is flat just
under the pelvis and ischial tuberosities, and then
slopes downward somewhat under the thighs.
Until such time this type of seat bottom may
become widely available, the preferred sitting
posture described below under "Recommendations"
will achieve decreased lumbar disc pressures
through full support of the lumbar lordosis.

An interesting method of quantifying the importance of the spinal contours, including the cervical
and lumbar lordosis, in their role of resisting the
compressive force of gravity is called the Delmas
Principle. This principle states that the spine's
ability to resist gravity (R) is equal to the square
of the number of normal spine contours present
(C^2) plus one (1), which can be expressed by the
equation $R = C^2 + 1$. *Proper sitting* as described in
this book supports the three normal spine contours
(cervical, thoracic, and lumbar); thus, the ability
of the spine to resist the compression of gravity
with good sitting posture can be expressed as
$R = 3^2 + 1 = 10$.

Improper sitting rounds out the normal contours of the lower back and neck as the pelvis tilts backward and the head pokes forward, leaving only the thoracic spine contour intact; thus, the ability of the spine to resist the compression of gravity with poor sitting posture can be expressed as $R = 1^2 + 1 = 2$. Comparing the relative values of 10 versus 2 numerically illustrates the spine's far greater ability to resist the compressive force of gravity with proper versus improper sitting posture.

Try to sit as correctly as possible at all times, but also remember that no one posture is the perfect posture because the body ultimately needs motion, and no one chair is the perfect design because how a person decides to sit in the chair determines its usefulness.

Recommendations

For working posture, The Science of Sitting recommends a seat with a cushioned surface and a "waterfall" (gradual sloping) seat edge. Avoid sitting on hard surfaces such plastic or metal stadium bleachers, concrete park benches, and wooden bar stools, or bring along your own seat cushion. The seat bottom of the chair may be slightly slanted downward from back to front a few degrees to assist forward rotation of the pelvis and slight opening of the thigh/trunk angle, but not so slanted as to cause sliding of the buttocks forward on the seat bottom. The back of the knees should not come into contact with the front edge of the seat bottom. The seatback should reach up to the top of the shoulder blades, be continuous without any large gaps, and be set to an upright (nearly vertical) position and locked in place. The lowest portion of the seatback ideally tapers away somewhat from the seat bottom to provide extra space for the buttocks as the mid and lower spine rest fully against the seatback. The point of greatest forward arch of the lumbar spine is where a lumbar support of 1—3" depth is ideally positioned. The correct chair height should allow the feet to contact the floor firmly with the knees at or below hip level. Armrests may be used if they do not restrict freedom of movement of the arms or forward travel of the chair toward the desk. The correct armrest level helps support the weight of the upper extremity without elevating the shoulders. Chairs that can swivel right and left as well as roll on the floor are preferred.

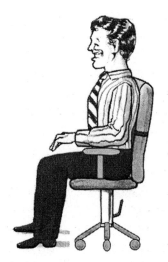

For resting posture, The Science of Sitting also recommends a cushioned surface and gradually sloping seat edges. The seat bottom of your chair need not be angled. The seatback should reach up to the back of the head and be continuous without any gaps, and may be set to any reclined position. The point of greatest forward arch of the lumbar spine is where a lumbar support is ideally positioned to fill that natural inward contour. The correct chair height should allow the feet to contact the floor firmly with the knees at or below hip level. An elevated footrest is optional to prop up the lower legs and feet. Armrests should help support the weight of the upper extremities without elevating the shoulders. Importantly, at all times while sitting in a reclined position, your head must stay in line with your mid and lower spine, well against the seatback or headrest, and not bent forward.

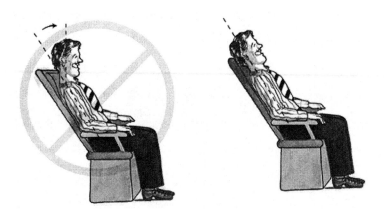

If one's posture is upright, one has no need to fear a crooked shadow.

Chinese proverb

F. Injury Prevention

Injuries at home or in the workplace can be painful to endure, expensive to manage, disabling in effect, and disruptive to life. The good news is that the great majority of injuries are completely avoidable with just a few moments of thinking before doing. Although the term "risk analysis" may sound complex, the practice of identifying hazards to prevent injury and save days, weeks, or months of undue suffering is actually very intuitive.

For example, would you suppose that lifting and carrying a 25-pound milk crate or a 25-pound sack of potatoes is more dangerous? The risk of injury would be greater lifting and carrying the sack of potatoes because its weight distribution is uneven and it is therefore more difficult to handle safely. Would you suppose that food preparation in a cold, dimly lit, and loud kitchen environment or a warm, brightly lit and sound moderated kitchen environment is more dangerous? The risk of injury would be greater in the cold, dimly lit, and overly noisy kitchen environment because the hand and eye coordination needed for cutting and chopping would be impaired by low temperature, poor lighting, and distracting noise levels.

These two examples illustrate that risk analysis is basically nothing more than common sense. Adding up the major risk factors to estimate the likelihood of injury for any particular task is as straightforward and predictable as $1 + 1 + 1 = 3$.

Most people consider injuries around the home, the workplace, and even out on the roadways to be "accidents." An accident by definition is both unintentional and unavoidable. We know for a fact that the great majority of household, work, and auto injuries are caused by poor judgment, unsafe practices, and/or inattention—all of which may be unintentional but are certainly avoidable. Therefore, most injuries are really no accident at all. By identifying and considering risk factors in advance, the opportunity to avoid injury for any particular activity becomes a matter of choice instead of just leaving it to chance.

You can apply this same method of risk analysis to those activities you participate in most often and surprise yourself with how much more you will learn about any particular activity no matter how long you have been doing it. If you have been injured in the past while on the job, performing a chore, or playing a sport, you can probably figure out why the injury occurred and how to prevent it from happening again.

Since lifting, deskwork, and repetitive motions are everyday activities for most people, let's look at some of the significant risk factors associated with each task. Once the major risk factors have been identified, it is simply a matter of minimizing them to the greatest extent possible, which will predictably reduce the risk of injury just as certainly as we know that $3 - 1 - 1 - 1 = 0$.

TASK: Lifting
Risk Factors:
1. Weight of the object
2. Size of the object
3. Distance of the object away from the mid-body
4. Lifting above shoulder or below knee level

1. As the weight of the object increases, the risk of injury increases from a) greater muscle effort needed to lift the load, and b) added compression of the weight on the discs and joints of the spine.

2. As the size of the object increases, the risk increases from a) holding the object further away from the body and b) awkward handholds and obstructed vision, causing more slips and falls.

3. As the distance of the object away from the mid-body increases (as with loading or unloading from the trunk of a car), the risk of injury rapidly increases from greater muscle effort needed to compensate for decreasing lifting leverage.

4. Lifting above shoulder level increases the risk of injury from greater muscle effort used by the smaller muscles of the shoulders and arms, and lifting below knee level increases the risk of injury from rounding the spine to bend down. Both also increase the risk of injury from greater object distance from the mid-body.

Example: Lifting a bag of dog food
Lifting a bag of dog food can be risky because the bags tend to be large and heavy and are typically stocked low to the ground. Reaching out to lift the bag places the load far forward of your body's center of gravity—a mechanical disadvantage. Advice: get help and make it a two-person lift.

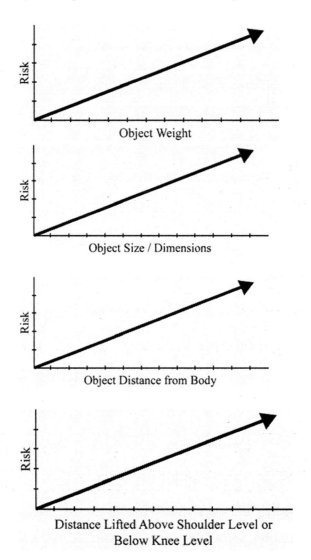

TASK: Seated Deskwork
Risk Factors:
1. Static posture
2. Turned or tilted head position
3. Rounding of the lower back
4. Shoulder elevation or arm reaching

1. The duration of continuous sitting without movement, called static posture, increases the risk of injury from prolonged tissue compression and lack of adequate blood flow.

2. The duration and the degree of head turning or tilting away from the neutral centered position increases the risk of injury from greater neck and upper back muscle effort needed to support the weight of the head.

3. The duration of lower back rounding out of the normal forward arch increases the risk of injury from greater disc compression and muscle effort needed to support the weight of the upper body.

4. The duration and degree of shoulder elevation or reaching out with the arm (often involved with keyboard and/or mouse use) increases the risk of injury from continuous muscle effort and the resultant decreased blood flow.

Example: data input
Sitting and working on a computer can put you at
risk because the task is highly sedentary for large
body parts but overactive for smaller body parts.
Often looking down or off to one side, or keeping
the shoulders raised, will make matters worse.
Advice: sit up properly and take frequent breaks.

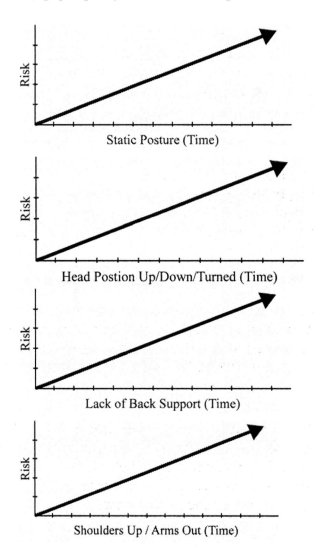

Static Posture (Time)

Head Postion Up/Down/Turned (Time)

Lack of Back Support (Time)

Shoulders Up / Arms Out (Time)

TASK: Repetitive Motions
Risk Factors:
1. Force or effort used
2. Number of repetitions
3. Range of movement
4. Rest periods (time)

1. Forceful activity that requires significant physical effort increases the risk of injury from greater strain on the muscles, joints, and connective tissues being used.

2. As the number of repetitions increases, so does the risk of injury from repeated use of the same group of muscles, joints, and connective tissues.

3. As the range of movement used for an activity increases in relation to the total motion possible for any body part, the risk of injury decreases as mechanical strain is spread out over a larger section of the body part during mobility.

4. As the frequency and/or duration of rest periods between bouts of activity increases, the risk of injury decreases with more recovery time.

Example: trimming hedges in a garden
Manual activity that requires firm grasping or arm strength against resistance can be a risk for Repetitive Motion Injury when the forces and reps are high and the motion and rest time are small, especially if you are unaccustomed to that activity. Advice: alternate heavy and light work in cycles.

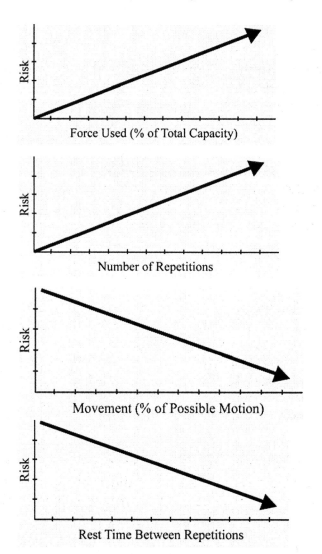

G. Winning the Battle with Back Pain

Back pain is very common. Most people will have a serious episode of back pain at some point in their lives. Many will have repeated episodes. Back pain can be quite disruptive to the daily routine of life, making even the simplest activity, such as sitting, standing, walking, or lying down comfortably a difficult task. If you twist an ankle, you can still get around reasonably well favoring your other leg to avoid using the injured side. But if you twist your back, getting around can be quite troublesome because it is almost impossible to avoid using your back.

The good news is that most people with back pain do recover. The question remains, how fast will you recover, and how completely? As painful and inconvenient as back pain can be, it seems worthwhile to do everything reasonable and necessary to assist the healing process and avoid more trouble down the road. Unfortunately, too many people unknowingly do the wrong things and don't do the right things in dealing with their back pain, which only prolongs the problem and diminishes the quality of healing.

Fortunately, the *need-to-know* information to avoiding and/or recovering from back pain is based on common sense, so it is easy to understand and act on. The following basic concepts should help you win the battle with most back pain episodes. Be sure to read through all eight sections, as each concept is interrelated with the others:

1. How Your Spine Works

Start by reviewing the fundamental parts and functions of your spine as described in Step One, Step Two, and "The Seated Spine" section of this book. It is important to know the normal shape of your spine, how it is held together, and how it works.

2. Pain On Purpose

Pain is a useful form of communication between you and your body. Pain usually means that something is being damaged or has already been damaged. People have most often ignored subtle hints of an impending problem before suffering a major back pain episode. The lesson here is, if you don't listen to your body when it whispers to you, your body will eventually get your attention by yelling at you. Instead of ignoring warning signs or dulling your senses to pain through over-medication, try to understand the message your body is sending you.

Pain is useful when it forces you to temporarily limit certain activities so that you avoid further injury. Pain can help you discover which body positions are better or worse for your particular back problem. Pain can remind you that you have been in one position too long. Pain can guide you to the directions of movement your body can best tolerate. Pain can help measure your improvement, or lack thereof, as your discomfort changes in line with the healing process.

Although you may be in a hurry to be completely out of pain, it is proper that you should feel better only when you actually are better. So take the time and the effort to do what is necessary to recover as fully and naturally as possible, so that pain-free actually means problem-free. Otherwise, it's only a matter of time before the next episode is triggered.

3. Knowing the Red Flags

A small percentage of the time, back pain can be a sign of a more serious underlying problem. Sometimes the intensity of pain is not as important as the location and the quality or nature of your symptoms. Common mechanical musculo-skeletal (muscle/joint)—type back pain can be very painful and disabling in the short-term, yet this type of pain is not usually considered to be as dangerous, for example, as an absence of sensation (numbness) or altered sensation (tingling). If you injure the muscles, joints, and/or connective tissue in your back and feel pain as a result, it means that your nerve system is functioning properly in communicating that message to you. However, if you feel no sensation or pain, or have altered sensations such as tingling or numbness, it means your nervous system is not functioning properly.

One type of pain that does raise a red flag is intractable pain; that is, pain without relief no matter what you do. If you cannot escape from your pain no matter what position you get in, despite the time of day or night, or regardless of the use of ice packs, muscle rubs, supports, and over-the-counter medication, you should seek professional help right away. Back pain with any of the following symptoms should also alert you that professional health care is urgently required:

Fever
Leg or arm weakness /coordination problems
Loss of bowel or bladder control
Loss of sensation (absence of any feeling)
Unintentional weight loss

Also be extra cautious if you have a health history of

Traumatic injury
Cancer
Osteoporosis
Long-term drug use (ex. corticosteroids)

The suggestions for managing back pain in this section will assume that you have none of the abovementioned red flags.

4. Timeframes for Healing

If you have a sudden onset of pain, there has usually been a strain of muscles and/or a sprain of connective tissues such as tendons, ligaments, joint capsules, and possibly discs (*the acute phase*). Strains and sprains cause small tears in the involved tissues and often result in pain, swelling, and reduced motion. Depending on the severity or degree of the injury, recovery from a strain/sprain may take a few days to a few months in total. However, the first few days following an acute injury—that is, the first 24—72 hours—are the most important and can set the stage for the remainder of the recovery.

After a few days or up to a week or so after an acute episode—again, depending on the degree of the strain and/or sprain—the repair process is ramping up and the body is mending the torn tissue fibers as best it can (*the subacute phase*). People that try to do too much, too soon at this timeframe often reinjure themselves and have to start over again with another acute episode. On the other hand, a complete lack of any motion or activity during this timeframe limits the speed and strength of the healing process. Most back pain episodes resolve during the subacute phase.

If pain or other symptoms such as stiffness or subjective weakness persist several weeks or months after the initial onset of a strain or sprain, the injury has likely mended with an inferior quality of tissue compared to the original structure, and muscular support has been weakened (*the chronic phase*). It is also possible that minor aggravating activities have repeatedly damaged the weakened structures so that you are caught in a perpetual reinjury/healing cycle. This cycle may not be broken until scar tissue adhesions are stripped away, weak tissue is strengthened, and/or aggravating activities (including ongoing postural strain) are avoided.

Note: Strictly maintaining good posture in your rest and activity positions to avoid reinjury is essential in all phases of back pain.

5. The Movement Prescription

In Step Nine of this book the importance of movement in maintaining health is explained. Body movement is beneficial in changing the position of joint surfaces, shifting tension of the connective tissues, and providing muscle contraction and lengthening, all of which increases circulation and fluid exchange—essentials for the healing process.

Immediately following a back injury or pain episode, in the *acute phase*, the best strategy is rest, support, and limited mobility. If every little movement you make is painful, just try to find the most comfortable stationary position. Often this position can be found by lying flat on your back with your knees elevated (as shown below), or on your side in a similar posture with a small pillow between your knees. Be sure to keep your head in a neutral position in line with your spine, not bent forward, and avoid sitting in any unsupported posture.

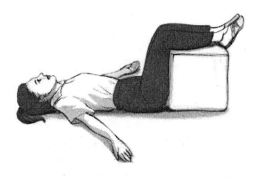

During the acute phase, an elastic back support can help compensate for some of the lost stability that is not being provided by the injured muscles, tendons, and ligaments, and can be worn almost continuously for up to 48 hours, except when bathing or performing the light movements described below. Within a few hours or days you should gain at least limited mobility in one direction or another.

When you are able to get into a hands and knees position on the floor, gently crawl forward using very small movements. You may also be able to perform the "cat-cow" yoga stretch, carefully and continuously raising and lowering your spine for about one minute exactly as shown, without changing the position of your arms and legs so that all of the motion comes from your back:

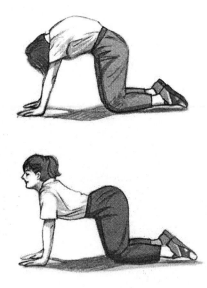

This is an excellent way to mobilize your spine without the vertical compression of gravity, as the stretch is performed with your back in a horizontal position. Movement and stretching after an injury or back pain episode should always be performed in a pain-free range of motion. That means you move only at the speed and to the extent that it causes no *further* pain.

At the time you can fully bear your own weight without the need for any elastic back support, and move better through a range of motion, you are probably in the *subacute phase*. Now is the time to facilitate the speed and quality of the healing process through mobility of the joints, muscles, and connective tissues. Walk short distances at a moderate pace on a flat surface. Try the stretches illustrated below. Perform the maneuvers on both sides of your body several times daily, and hold each position ten seconds.

a. Standing side stretch

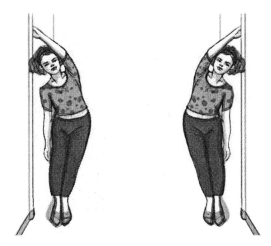

b. Lying knee-to-opposite-shoulder stretch

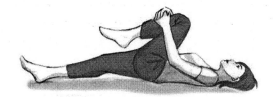

c. Alternating arm/leg extension exercise

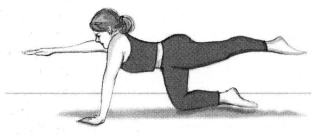

These three basic stretching exercise positions take your spine through all the planes of motion: flexion, extension, side-bending, and rotation. If you can minimize aggravating movements and positions, but gain more strength and flexibility through walking and stretching exercises, you should be able to work your way through the healing process and resolve the back pain episode.

After several weeks or months, if pain or other symptoms remain, you are likely in a *chronic phase* and may benefit from professional help with formal evaluation for specific exercise, stretch, and ergonomics advice or physical rehabilitation recommendations. The "natural course" of back pain is resolution after a few days or weeks (which can be significantly speeded up or slowed down by what you do, or do not do, in earlier phases). When symptoms do not resolve as expected, the exact obstacle(s) to healing must be identified and overcome on an individual basis.

6. Ice or Heat?

Temperature changes can assist the healing process and beneficially affect the spine and its supportive structures if used correctly. The intent is to flush the injured area with blood flow, like the rising and falling of the ocean tide, to facilitate delivery of oxygen and nutrition and the removal of metabolic waste products. The difference between ice and heat is the way they are used to increase circulation. Ice initially directs blood flow away from the area where it's applied. Heat initially directs blood flow into the area where it's applied.

The *acute phase* of a back episode usually involves new or greater pain and a degree of swelling, which is an accumulation of fluids and heat. Therefore, ice is the best choice to first direct blood flow away. Depending on the thickness of the area, a 15—20 minute application is generally sufficient and also produces a local analgesic (pain-reducing) effect. The ice pack should then be removed from the skin and the area allowed to return to normal body temperature. This process is then repeated throughout the day. In this way, circulation is increased by repeatedly drawing blood flow away from the injured area, then drawing it back upon removal of the ice pack as rewarming of the area occurs.

The *chronic phase* of a back episode often involves symptoms of stiffness, subjective weakness, and a certain baseline level of on-going pain. Scarring of connective tissue or tightened muscles may result in a decrease of circulation to the injured area. Therefore, heat is the best choice to direct blood flow into the affected area first. Depending on the thickness of the area, a 15—20 minute application is usually sufficient and also produces a relaxing effect.   The heat should then be removed from the skin and the area allowed to return to normal body temperature. This process is then repeated. In this way, circulation is increased by repeatedly drawing blood into the affected area, then having it disperse upon removal of the heat as cooling of the area occurs.

The *subacute phase* of a back episode usually represents an improvement over the acute phase in terms of symptoms and physical function. However, this stage can relapse into an acute phase if the partially healed area of the spine is provoked through reinjury, or can proceed into a chronic phase if the healing process stalls. So, during the subacute phase, a combination of ice application, then heat application, repeated over several cycles is the best choice to direct blood flow away from and then back into the affected area. After each ice or heat application, wait for the body area to return to a normal skin temperature before switching to the next application.

7. Professional Help

There are a number of different health care professionals that work with people suffering from back pain, including medical physicians (general and specialty practice, including osteopaths), physical therapists, chiropractors, acupuncturists, massage therapists, athletic trainers, and exercise physiologists. When is the right time to visit a professional for help with back pain, and which type of practitioner should you choose? The answer may vary from person to person, but in no instance should a person with any of the red flags mentioned earlier delay in seeking professional help. Urgent health care situations aside, there are more choices and considerations in deciding when to go and whom to see.

Regarding when to go, people with little knowledge about appropriate self-care measures during a back pain episode would be well served by getting some professional advice to help shorten their episode or avoid becoming a chronic case. Those with back pain more uncomfortable than they are willing to bear, slower healing than they would consider reasonable, or with fairly consistent recurrent episodes, are also good candidates for professional analysis and treatment.

Regarding whom to see, it is worth mentioning that although there are few certainties when it comes to dealing with back pain in our society, one thing for sure is that no one type of practitioner can help every type of patient. Perhaps that explains why there are so many different approaches to back pain problems. When seeking professional help, it is usually a good idea to ask friends, family, co-workers, or another health care provider if they can recommend someone with a good reputation. Even though the different back care professionals have some distinct ideologies and use some different methods, the most important consideration is that they are good at their particular discipline.

Here is a basic rundown of the different health care professionals and some of the treatment tools they often use:

medical physicians (medication, injections, surgery, and osteopathic manipulation)
physical therapists (physical therapy modalities, physical rehabilitation, soft tissue and joint mobilization, and ergonomics advice)
chiropractors (chiropractic adjustment, physiotherapy, soft tissue work, exercise, stretching, ergonomics and nutritional advice)
acupuncturists (acupuncture, acupressure, and herbal medicine)
massage therapists (soft tissue work)
athletic trainers and exercise physiologists (physical rehabilitation)

Some of the more common diagnostic testing that may be ordered by a health care professional to assess your back pain include:

plain film x-rays
MRI/CT (high resolution in multiple planes)
EMG/NCV (muscle and nerve conduction tests)

There are many other special tests available, but they are not as commonly utilized. Biofeedback and psychology are two additional specialties that may be considered in certain back pain cases because stress significantly worsens back pain.

Although you can rely on most health care professionals for their expertise and advice, you cannot delegate away your need to understand your condition and to consent to any proposed treatment plan. Below is a list of important questions to ask your doctor or therapist about back pain. First be prepared to offer the following basic information to help your doctor or therapist correctly assess your problem:

Where it hurts
What the symptoms feel like
When it started
If it has happened before
How often it hurts
What aggravates or relieves the pain

Then, after your assessment and before any treatment, your doctor or therapist should clearly explain to you the answers to the following questions:

1. What seems to be the problem?
2. What is the most likely cause of the problem?
3. What parts of the body are involved?
4. Does the problem involve one or more spinal levels, right or left side, centralized?
5. Are there any more tests that could help further identify the problem?
6. What treatment is recommended?

7. Will this treatment resolve the cause of the problem?

8. How long will the treatment take and is there a recovery period involved?

9. Is the treatment expected to improve how I feel and how I function?

10. What are the risks of treatment and the possible consequences of not being treated?

8. Dietary Recommendations

You need basic nutrition to assist the healing process, and you need to avoid substances that will impede your recovery. Basic nutrition comes from a balance of complex carbohydrates, lean proteins, and unsaturated fats. There are many resources available to help you find good sources of these food components. Try to eat food that is grown or raised, such as vegetables, fruits, legumes, whole grains, raw nuts, beef, fish, and fowl, lightly prepared and close to its natural state, because heavily modified foods have far less fiber, vitamins, and minerals.

In most instances, real, fresh, raw food has fewer calories and more nutrients, while processed, packaged, preserved food has more calories and fewer nutrients. Moderate caffeine and avoid smoking, alcohol, and any unnecessary medication, as these can impair your normal circulation, hydration, and metabolism. Finally, how much you eat and your total body composition will also weigh heavily on current and future health issues.

Summary

Acute Phase: ice, rest (flat back and knees elevated), support and limited mobility ("cat-cow" yoga stretch/gentle crawling)

Subacute Phase: alternate ice and heat, gradually increase activity, mobility, and strength (walking, standing arm-over-head side stretch, lying on your back knee-to-opposite-shoulder stretch, and alternating leg extension exercise)

Chronic Phase: heat, continue non-aggravating activity, stretch and exercise, identify exact obstacle(s) to healing such as ongoing postural faults, scar tissue, weakness

Remember good posture practice throughout all phases of healing to help avoid reinjury!

Notes Section

About the Author

Gregg J. Carb attended the University of California, Irvine and California State University, Northridge before entering the Cleveland College of Chiropractic in Los Angeles. He graduated cum laude in 1985 with a B.S. in Human Biology and a D.C. (Doctor of Chiropractic). Additional professional qualifications include appointments by the State of California as a Qualified Medical Evaluator for workers' compensation and as an Independent Medical Examiner for state disability, and certification as an Associate Ergonomist by the Oxford Research Institute. Dr. Carb is also a certified ART® (Active Release Techniques) provider for repetitive strain and athletic injuries, and maintains a clinical practice in San Francisco, California.

Dr. Carb's interest in posture and ergonomics is a natural extension of the chiropractic emphasis on the relationship between anatomical structure and physiological function and of more than twenty years of practice working with a diverse patient population ranging from computer programmers to triathletes. Time, training, and experience have all shown him that when it comes to health, aging, and fitness—*posture matters*.

The success of the first and second editions of his *Sitting Pretty* books have inspired Dr. Carb to greatly expand and enhance the content of his earlier work while maintaining a focus on helping people understand and improve what they are doing most often throughout the day—sitting.

Glossary

Abdomen—Belly area between the chest and pelvis

Bone deposits—Irregular growths above and beyond normal bone margins

Cervical—Spine region in the neck

Deformity—A change from the normal shape

Degeneration—Wear-and tear-breakdown that usually causes hardening and rigidity

Ergonomics—The science of human interaction with objects and/or processes

Kyphosis—Backward arch of the spine found in the mid-back (kyphotic curve)

Lordosis—Forward arch of the spine found in the neck and lower back (lordotic curve)

Lumbar—Spine region in the lower back

Neutral position—Body posture that maintains the normal shape of the spine

Primary curve—Kyphotic curve of the mid-back

Secondary curve—Lordotic curves of the neck and lower back

Sedentary—Inactive; often refers to sitting

Slumping—Poor sitting or standing posture characterized by drooping or slouching

Spine—The "backbone" or spinal column, made of twenty-four vertebrae; seven in the neck, twelve in the mid-back, and five in the lower back; plus the sacrum (base) and coccyx (tailbone)

Static posture—One position held without motion

Scar tissue—Dense fibrous connective tissue that replaces healthy tissue after injury or damage

Thoracic—Spine region in the mid-back

Thorax—Chest area between the head and belly

Vertebrae—Spinal bones; singular is vertebra

Vertically aligned—Straight up and down

Bibliography

1. Looze MP, et al. Sitting comfort and discomfort and the relationship with objective measures. Ergonomics 2003: 46(10).

2. Cagnie B. et al. Individual and work related risk factors for neck pain among office workers: a cross sectional study. Eur Spine J Dec 8 2006.

3. Schwab F, Dubey A, et al. Adult scoliosis: A health assessment analysis by SF-36. Spine 2003: 28(6).

4. Martin-Du Pan R. et al. The role of body position and gravity in the symptoms and treatment of various medical diseases. Swiss Med Wkly 2004; 134:543-551.

5. Stokes I. et al. Influence of the Hamstring Muscles on Lumbar Spine Curvature in Sitting. Spine 1980; Vol 5 No. 6, 525-528.

6. Lennon J., Shealy C., Cady R., Matta W., Cox R., Simpson W. Postural and Respiratory Modulation of Autonomic Function, Pain, and Health. AJPM 1994; 4:36-39.

7. Bridger R., Von Eisenhart-Rothe C., Henneberg M. Effects of Seat Slope and Hip Flexion on Spinal Angles. Human Factors 1989; 31(6): 679-688.

8. Rempel D., Wang P., Janowitz P., Harrison R., Yu F, Ritz B. A Randomized Controlled Trial Evaluating the Effects of New Task Chairs on Shoulder and Neck Pain Among Sewing Machine Operators. Spine 2007; 32(9): 931-938.

9. Saarini L., Nygard C., Rimpela A., Nummi T., Kaukiainen A. The Working Postures Among Schoolchildren – A Controlled Intervention Study on the Effects of Newly Designed Workstations. Journal of School Health 2007; 77(5): 240-247.

Index

Acupuncturists, 165, 166
Anterior head carriage, 139
Arthritis, 134, 137
Athletic trainers, 165, 166

Biofeedback, 167
Bookmark/monitor placard, 119, 126
Breathing, deep, 81, 128, 129

Cat-cow yoga stretch, 160, 169
Chiropractors 165, 166
Curves, primary, 25
Curves, secondary, 25

Dehydration, 46, 137
Deformity, 15, 33, 34, 61, 72, 113
Degeneration, 15, 35-37, 61, 112, 117, 134
Delmas principle, 141
Deskwork, seated, 81, 150
Diagnostic testing, 166
Dowager's hump, 34

Ergonomic devices, 63, 113
Ergonomic tune-up, 96, 102
Ergonomic tune-up checklist, 102
Exercise, alternating arm/leg, 162, 169
Exercise physiologists, 165, 166
Eyestrain, 103

Footrest, 54, 57, 64, 98, 118, 144
Forward head posture, 50, 72

Healing, timeframes, 157
Heat, 131, 163, 164, 169

Ice, 163, 164, 169
Insole, 104
Isometric contraction, 37

Kyphosis, 34

Lever arm, 138
Lifting, 89, 108, 138, 148, 149
Lying flat, 159

Massage therapists, 165, 166

Neutral position, 18, 29, 39, 40, 71, 88, 112, 113, 159
Notes section, 18, 170
Nutrition, 163, 168

Office furniture, 66
Osteopaths, 165
Osteoporosis, 34, 157

Physical therapists, 165, 166
Physicians, medical, 165,166
Pillow, 70, 72, 93, 95, 106, 159
Posture awareness, 13, 18, 59, 61, 62, 88
Posture habits, 17, 18, 33, 34, 42, 60, 62, 63, 65, 112
Posture, resting, 88, 135, 144
Posture restoration, 15
Posture, static, 18, 150
Posture tips, 89
Posture, working, 135, 141, 142
Psychology, 167

Red flags, 156, 157, 165
Repetitive motions, 38, 63, 147, 152
Repetitive strain injuries, 74
Risk analysis, 146, 147

Scapulae, 48
Scar tissue, 36-38, 158, 169
Sedentary, 19, 86, 94, 151
Self-Care Record, 64, 127, 129, 130
Sit bones, 25, 84, 140
Sit disc, 75, 82, 128
Slumping, compression effect, 54
Stress, 69, 128, 129, 167
Stretch, hamstring, 84

Stretch, knee-to-opposite-shoulder, 162, 169
Stretch, range of motion, 80, 128
Stretch, standing side, 161, 169

Thigh/trunk angle, 140, 142
Traction, 68

Vertically align(ed), 22, 40, 56
Video games, 94

Workout, sixty second, 75, 76, 127, 129

For book order information, posture research, downloadable documents, updates, and more, please visit www.scienceofsitting.com